Luminos is the Open Access monograph publishing program from UC Press. Luminos provides a framework for preserving and reinvigorating monograph publishing for the future and increases the reach and visibility of important scholarly work. Titles published in the UC Press Luminos model are published with the same high standards for selection, peer review, production, and marketing as those in our traditional program. www.luminosoa.org

The publisher and the University of California Press Foundation gratefully acknowledge the generous support of the Ahmanson Foundation Endowment Fund in Humanities.

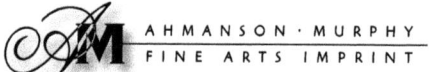

THE AHMANSON FOUNDATION has endowed this imprint to honor the memory of FRANKLIN D. MURPHY who for half a century served arts and letters, beauty and learning, in equal measure by shaping with a brilliant devotion those institutions upon which they rely.

The Erotics of History

The Erotics of History

An Atlantic African Example

Donald L. Donham

UNIVERSITY OF CALIFORNIA PRESS

University of California Press, one of the most distinguished university presses in the United States, enriches lives around the world by advancing scholarship in the humanities, social sciences, and natural sciences. Its activities are supported by the UC Press Foundation and by philanthropic contributions from individuals and institutions. For more information, visit www.ucpress.edu.

University of California Press
Oakland, California

© 2018 by Donald L. Donham

Suggested citation: Donham, D. L. *The Erotics of History: An Atlantic African Example.* Oakland: University of California Press, 2018.
doi: https://doi.org/10.1525/luminos.45

This work is licensed under a Creative Commons CC-BY-NC-ND license. To view a copy of the license, visit http://creativecommons.org/licenses.

Library of Congress Cataloging-in-Publication Data

Names: Donham, Donald L. (Donald Lewis), author.
Title: The erotics of history : an Atlantic African example / Donald L. Donham.
Description: Oakland, California : University of California Press, [2018] | Includes bibliographical references and index.
Identifiers: LCCN 2017044673 | ISBN 9780520296312 (pbk.)
Subjects: LCSH: Fetishism (Sexual behavior)--Africa--History. | Erotica--Africa--History. | Sex role--Africa--History. | Africa--Sexual behavior--History. | Africa--Social conditions--History.
Classification: LCC HQ79 .D57 2018 | DDC 305.3096--dc23
LC record available at https://lccn.loc.gov/2017044673

When I think about fetishism I want to know about many other things. I do not see how one can talk about fetishism, or sadomasochism, without thinking about the production of rubber, the techniques and gear used for controlling and riding horses, the high polished gleam of military footwear, the history of silk stockings, the cold authoritative qualities of medical equipment, or the allure of motorcycles and the elusive liberties of leaving the city for the open road. For that matter, how can we think of fetishism without the impact of cities, of certain streets and parks, of red-light districts and "cheap amusements," or the seductions of department store counters, piled high with desirable and glamorous goods . . . ? To me, fetishism raises all sorts of issues concerning shifts in the manufacture of objects, the historical and social specificities of control and skin and social etiquette, or ambiguously experienced body invasions and minutely graduated hierarchies.
 —Gayle Rubin, "*Sex Traffic*"

Nothing is as it seems. History is carried like a pathology, a cyclical melodrama immersed in artifice and unable to function without it. The historical romance creates a will for abusive submission, exacerbated by contemporary ideologies that revere victimhood. Everyone wants to play the nigger now.
 —Kara E. Walker, *Look Away! Look Away! Look Away!*

CONTENTS

List of Illustrations xi

Preface xiii

Heading South: An Introduction
1

1. Ethnography Interruptus
18

2. The Concept of the Fetish
28

3. African Origins
33

4. The Poverty of Sexuality
43

5. African Sexual Extraversion and Getting into Bed with Robert Mapplethorpe
50

6. Para-ethnography, Golf, and the Internet
59

7. White Slavery
65

8. Love and Money, Romance and Scam
78

Conclusion: Toward an Understanding of Erotics
83

Notes 101
Bibliography 113
Index 133

ILLUSTRATIONS

1. *Terra del fuoco* (Land of Fire), by Baron Wilhelm von Gloeden 2
2. Leni Riefenstahl in the Nuba Mountains 6
3. *Ragazzo con pesce volante* (Boy with a Flying Fish), by Baron Wilhelm von Gloeden 17
4. A Kongo *nkisi*, by an unknown carver 37
5. A sketch from a photograph of a white slave working in an African field 68

PREFACE

It is properly ironic that an anthropologist who has spent most of his career extolling the virtues of ethnography should be brought up, finally, against the advantages of leaving it behind—at least for a time. After the reader has put down this book, questions will remain with regard to the social and cultural life of the African neighborhood I describe. Perhaps one day, in a different political climate, they can be answered more fully.

What I hope to accomplish is, rather, the construction of a theoretical approach that will effectively problematize the case under review—an example of white gay European males traveling to West Africa in search of black male lovers (most of whom are married or soon to be married to African women). Starting from this instance, my goal is to assemble the theoretical resources for an approach to the erotic that does not exceptionalize my materials. I argue that the concept of "sexuality" implicitly proceeds from a standpoint that accepts "heterosexuality" as a standard from which deviations from the norm are measured and defined.

In place of sexuality, I begin with the concept of the fetish. What was, in the nineteenth century, a way of explaining the sexual margins is, in my exposition, the base of *all* sexual excitement—even, or especially, for so-called straight persons. The notion of the fetish extends far beyond sexual matters and is a part of an exceptionally long and deep conversation in social theory about how persons and things constitute one another. For my purposes, I start by juxtaposing Marx and Freud. Étienne Balibar has recently argued that over the course of Marx's development, the fetish replaced ideology as the fulcrum of his economic philosophy. And Michel Foucault pointed out some time ago that fetishism was the "model perversion" for nineteenth- and early twentieth-century sexual scientists, up to Freud. I take this conversation up to the present in relation to Bruno Latour's notion of the "factish."[1]

With respect to Western notions of sex, I have taught, for many years, an undergraduate course called Sexualities. Yet, the longer I have taught the course, the more convinced I have become of the descriptive inadequacy of the notion of sexualities. This has occurred while my students have, in contrast, embraced the notion ever more fervently. After the enormous influence of Foucault's *The History of Sexuality, Vol. 1,* and then near three decades of queer theory, what is going on?

On the African side, the challenges are greater. One of the dominant sites for the construction of Western racism has always involved sex, particularly notions of excessive and/or deviant sex. How does one examine African erotics without seeming to play into racist notions? That quandary has, no doubt, helped to inhibit the study of the erotic in Africa. This vacuum has allowed some Africans in the last decade to adopt the Western discourse on sexuality with a vengeance. African heterosexuality has become pure, uncontaminated African tradition, while homosexuality, in contrast, has become an unnatural import from the West. Some African nationalists in Uganda, for example, have recently gone so far as to propose the death penalty for local "homosexuals."

Examining the erotic, anywhere, inevitably holds the potential for trespassing readers' (differing) views of where analysis slides into voyeurism. And in the case under review, sex, race, and politics are tied together in an unusually tight knot. My goal is slowly to untie that knot to reveal the complex ways that fantasies of various sorts interact with and sometimes create local social realities. What constitutes a sex-positive analysis in the West, much less in Africa, is, of course, a contested question. I offer, in this book, one answer.

Each of my books has reflected the context of a particular department, a specific network of friends and interlocutors. *The Erotics of History* is my University of California book. First of all, I want to thank my many colleagues in the Department of Anthropology at UC Davis, who have read and commented on multiple drafts.

I began this work in the fall of 2012 while I was a fellow at the University of California Humanities Research Institute at UC Irvine. I thank Kalindi Vora and Neda Atanasoski for their roles in organizing our group and other members for feedback and inspiration. Afterward, a Berkeley discussion group—organized by Mariane Ferme—provided a continuing sounding board. And an early version of this work was presented to the Department of Anthropology at Duke University in the fall of 2014. I thank Engseng Ho for the invitation and members of the department for stimulating feedback.

A Gallery for Fine Photography in New Orleans put me in contact with Joel-Peter Witkin, whose 2012 photograph *Penis*

High Heel Shoe With Turnips, New Mexico appears on the cover. Finally, and perhaps most importantly, I want to thank San Franciscans Lisa Rofel and Gayle Rubin for their support and critical comment.

This book is dedicated to "Johnny," my erstwhile Oakland neighbor without whom it could never have been written. To thank any of these individuals does not imply, of course, that they necessarily agree with the analysis that follows.

Oakland, California

Heading South

An Introduction

For over two centuries now, privileged northern European men have traveled to Mediterranean lands in search of male-male sex and love. Pushed by social rejection, scandal, and sometimes executions, and pulled by travelers' reports of more relaxed southern mores[1]—and, ironically, by censorious descriptions of the acceptance of "unnatural vice" in Islamic lands—European men were drawn into a long conversation of acts and ideas.

Early twentieth-century German sexologist Iwan Bloch (1933, 31) must have reflected popular opinion when he wrote: "It can, indeed, be due only to climatic conditions that today sexual perversions, especially homosexuality, are more deep-rooted, more frequent, and much less severely judged by the public morality in southern Europe than in northern; that in fact there are great differences between northern and southern Italy in this respect."

Bloch seems to have been echoing Sir Richard Burton's late nineteenth-century creation of what the latter termed the Sotadic Zone—a band across the globe that extended from the

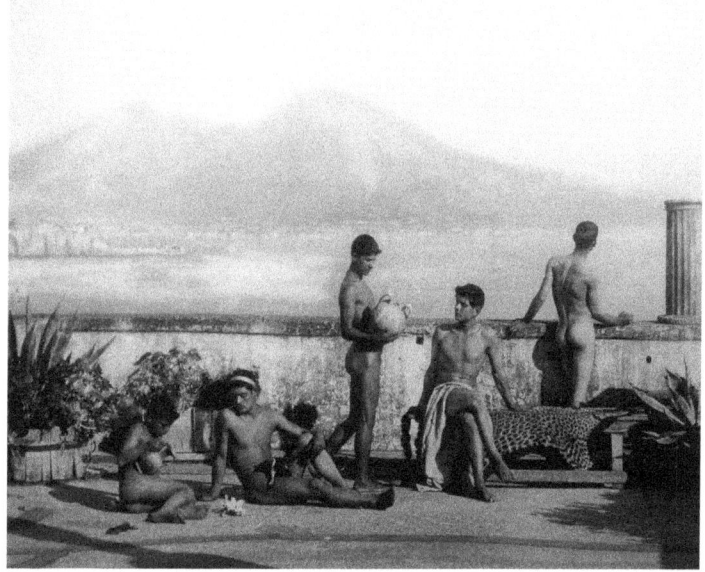

Figure 1. *Terra del fuoco* (Land of Fire), by Baron Wilhelm von Gloeden. One of von Gloeden's most famous images, it captures Vesuvius from a terrace in Naples. The south is a land of warmth and pleasure in which unexpected desires can erupt.

Mediterranean eastward through the Middle East to China and Japan to the preconquest New World, in which, according to Burton, male same-sex sex was "popular and endemic, held at the worst to be a mere peccadillo, whilst the races to the North and South of its limits... practice it only sporadically amid the opprobrium of their fellows who, as a rule, are physically incapable of performing the operation and look upon it with the liveliest disgust" (quoted in Bleys 1995, 217).

It was not, of course, that Mediterranean cultures were somehow "looser"; they were simply differently structured.[2] Extending back to ancient Greece (Halperin 1990), what was prohibited for adult men was not simply other men but being penetrated by other men. Thus, it often appeared to upper-class northerners that virtually *any* Sicilian or Arab was available to them, but, of course, the terms of that availability were nonetheless structured.³

By the 1890s, photographic images of young Mediterranean male bodies began to encourage traffic to the south. Figure 1 was made into postcards by Wilhelm von Gloeden, a Prussian nobleman who had settled in the Sicilian town of Taormina. It broadly invokes ancient Greece (always in the background of the educated European imagination of male-male sex). The combination of fantasy and political economy extends into the present in what we now call, somewhat reductively, sex tourism.

Von Gloeden evidently had sexual relationships with many of his photographic models.

> It is interesting to consider the manner in which that small Sicilian town dealt with the knowledge of Guglielmo Gloeden's sexual proclivities, for it is certain that many people knew of them . . . It is noteworthy that some of his most constant supporters were the simplest women of the town: an egg seller, washer women, fish wives. A clue to this loyalty is found in a fact little known even to his close friends. Von Gloeden had not infrequently provided the dowries for the daughters of poor families whose suitors were young men of whom von Gloeden was fond. (Leslie 1977, 42–44)

The north-south interchange began well before the consolidation of the European idea of homosexuality. Thus in England in 1809, after a spurt of hanging and pillorying of men accused of sodomy, Lord Byron set out on his first journey to Ottoman Greece. Enamored of both young men and women, Byron may have been drawn to Islamic lands by his reading of translations of Persian classical poets with similar attractions (Crompton 1985, 111–29). Staying in a monastery in Athens, Byron developed a relationship with a young man, Niccolo Giraud, serious enough that he would include the latter, at one point, in his will (Crompton 1985, 146–57). On his way home, Byron enrolled Giraud in a school on Malta, after which we lose track of this young man. Speaking Greek, Italian, and English, did Giraud become a successful businessman in a Mediterranean world pulled ever closer into the economic orbit of northern Europe?

Many others followed in Byron's steps: the Hanoverian lawyer Karl Heinrich Ulrichs, in many ways the world's first queer activist;[4] perhaps the philosopher Friedrich Nietzsche (Köhler 2002); the British adventurer T. E. Lawrence; and a myriad of creative writers, including Oscar Wilde, André Gide, E. M. Forster, William Burroughs, and Joe Orton (Boone 2014; Aldrich 2003; Mullins 2002). In 1968, French philosopher Michel Foucault missed some of the iconic events of the uprising in Paris because he was living in Sidi Bou Saïd, teaching at the University of Tunis (Macey 1993, 181–208).

Finally, Americans Paul and Jane Bowles settled in Tangier just after World War II. In anticipation of anthropologists' enthusiasm for collaborative ethnography after the 1980s, Paul Bowles began transcribing stories from Moroccan men in the 1960s—many his lovers—listing himself only as translator: Mohammed Mrabet's *Love with a Few Hairs* and Larbi Layachi's *A Life Full of Holes* both explore the interrelationship between European-Moroccan, male-male love and the local forms of male-female marriage that the former underwrote and made possible.

After two hundred years, much has changed in these interactions. As homosexual identity—and therefore heterosexuality—became more totalizing in the United States after World War II, many straight-identified men would no longer have sex with men, in any form. According to Hilderbrand (2013), gay travel from North America by the 1970s was, to some extent, a search for foreign social scenes less affected by this cultural transformation, ones in which North American gay men could still have sex with straight men, "trade" they sometimes paid.

There were changes on the other side of the north/south interaction as well. By the early twentieth century, uncolonized Islamic lands like Persia, the elites of which had become intensely aware of Western repudiation of their sexual customs, quickly gave up long-established patterns of male-male love in their strivings to become "modern" (Najmabadi 2005). Apparently, nothing transforms sexual cultures as effectively as the mobilization of shame and embarrassment,[5] so much so that now many in Islamic lands and sub-Saharan Africa know nothing of their same-sex sexual prehistories.[6] As I have said, "homosexuality" is assumed by many in these areas to be a uniquely Western preoccupation.

In this essay, I take up the analysis of a case that continues older Mediterranean patterns but situates them in the different cultural context of Atlantic Africa after decolonization. A central part of European male fantasy that I have just described involved the attribution of extramasculinity to Sicilian and Arab men. But if so, African men were and continue to be doubly submitted to this regime, as Frantz Fanon argued years ago in *Black Skin, White Masks* ([1952] 2008).

In such a context, it is perhaps not surprising that the major streams of recent sex tourism to Africa have involved European women traveling south in search of African men (on such patterns in West Africa, see Ebron 1997; in East Africa, Meiu 2008, 2017). These interactions are now mediated not only by books and photographs but also by the Internet and its dating websites. And these more recent forms of communication have led

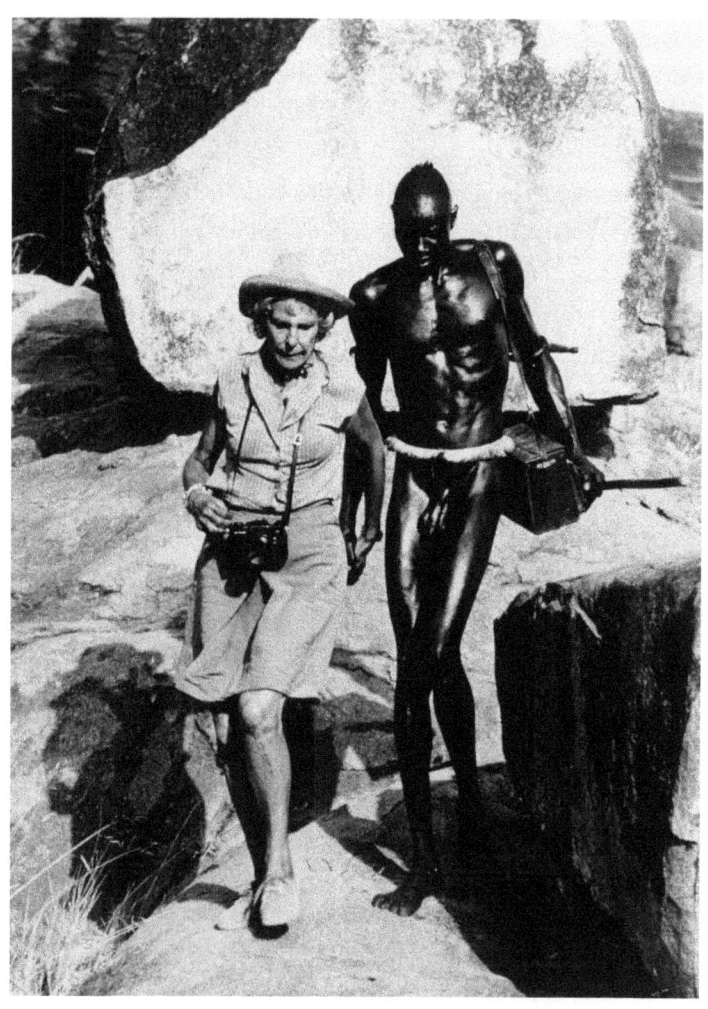

Figure 2. Leni Riefenstahl in the Nuba Mountains, courtesy of Getty Images (Keystone/Hulton Archive).

to the explosion of what are now called romance scams. The FBI recently estimated that in 2015 alone such schemes netted more than $200 million from North Americans.[7]

But of course masculinity has also been an attraction for some European men. Without what Europeans regarded, and many still regard, as the civilizational attainments that Arabs had—a past tradition of monumental architecture, written languages, historical records, world religions—African men appeared closer to nature and therefore as enticingly, and sometimes threateningly, supersexed. When the memory of massive European enslavement of West African populations is added to this mix, an especially complex erotic field is created—as African American artist Kara Walker (1995), black British filmmaker Isaac Julien (1994), and black gay literary theorists like Robert Reid-Pharr (2001) and Darieck Scott (2010) have begun to explore.

As I shall show below, sadomasochism or SM, a controversial practice within gay networks of the great Western cities after the 1950s, became a part of the African scene I am going to describe. SM was, among other things, a quest for masculine styles. Ironically, the logic of racialization tended to place African men in the role of tops in SM fantasies. This inversion of the actual historical pattern—accompanied by the fantasy that the upending was motivated by black revenge for past white oppression—created a particular erotic experience for both Europeans and Africans.[8] Inversely, when African men less frequently became servants or slaves in SM scenes, the historical verisimilitude must have added an edgy, dangerous frisson. Either way, there was no escaping history.

My focus is on, then, what I'm calling the erotics of history, how peculiar erotic attachments of individuals are conditioned by wider historical and cultural patterns and memories. For an extraordinarily well-documented example of this connection—and for an illustration of why such intimate details are usually so difficult to obtain—see Davidoff (1974, 1979). Davidoff describes the case of a late nineteenth-century English gentleman, Arthur Munby, who obsessively documented what we would now call a consensual SM relationship with a domestic maid, Hannah Cullwick, whom Munby secretly married (but with whom he never had sexual intercourse). Both Munby and Cullwick left diaries, photographs, and drawings that Munby willed to the archives of Trinity College, Cambridge. It was almost as if this documentation had become a fetish in itself. It recalled and reenacted sexual excitement. Following Anne McClintock's impressive *Imperial Leather* (1995), which reanalyzed the Munby-Cullwick case, especially in relation to colonial themes, I would like to situate stories of sexual attraction—fetishes—within the wider contours and changes of postcolonial capitalism itself.[9]

To be able to accomplish that, I have found that I must reject a persistent conceptual move made over the last few decades involving what seems to me to be the attribution of an illusory power to the concept of sexuality: that is, that sexualities are consistent states of being, relatively stable forms of personhood, that stand behind and produce, cause, and organize erotic attachments. That the same person can, for example, feel quite different erotic attractions in different contexts, that social forces like peer pressure, both negative and positive, can be transformative, and that erotic commitments can change, sometimes significantly so—all these are elided. Despite the fluidity that results, the notion of sexuality seems somehow protected as an essence or a condition, whether it is thought to be biologically or culturally constituted.[10]

I am hardly the first to make this argument. Consider how far back the position I advocate goes, well before queer theory:[11] "It would encourage clearer thinking on these matters if persons were not characterized as heterosexual or homosexual, but as individuals who have had certain amounts of heterosexual experience and certain amounts of homosexual experience. Instead of using these terms as substantives which stand for persons, or even as adjectives to describe persons, they may better be used to describe the nature of the overt sexual relations, or of the stimuli to which an individual erotically responds" (Kinsey, Pomeroy, and Martin 1948, 617).[12]

At one point, Kinsey et al. anticipated what is called labeling theory, developed by sociologists in the 1960s:

> One of the factors that materially contributes to the development of exclusively homosexual histories, is the ostracism which society imposes upon one who is discovered to have had perhaps no more than a lone experience. The high school boy is likely to be expelled from school and, if it is in a small town, he is almost certain to be driven from the community. His chances of making heterosexual contacts are tremendously reduced after the public disclosure, and he is forced into the company of other homosexual individuals among whom he finally develops an exclusively homosexual pattern for himself. (Kinsey, Pomeroy, and Martin 1948, quoted in Plummer 1981, 17–18)

The opposition between heterosexuality and homosexuality critiqued by Kinsey et al. depends fundamentally on the categorical oppositions created when the biological reproduction of human beings is assumed as a master teleology—heterosexual versus homosexual, straight versus queer, the second term being always the assumed reproductive failure.

The problem is that nonreproductive sex seems universally present in human societies, is institutionalized in many cases, and is even celebrated in a few. And its presence may be, I shall suggest, currently increasing. Of course, biological reproduction must be effected at some level for societies and cultures to persist. But with respect to any particular society, this reproduction does not have to occur through biological means (see Paul 2015 for examples). The teleology, if there is one, is social and cultural reproduction—processes that can, in fact, contradict genetic evolutionary logic.[13] I would argue, then, that we begin to think of the erotic as establishing the attractions required by sociality itself—one by-product of which can be biological reproduction.[14]

Without biological reproduction as the master teleology, the separation of object choice—from any number of other possibilities when it comes to the erotic—no longer makes sense. Now the question becomes, what is it about cultural definitions and individual and group memories that underlie what have been called fetishes that makes sex sexy?

Given my argument, wouldn't it be clarifying to throw out the entire apparatus of sexuality? The problem with such a move is that some social actors themselves, "homosexuals," decades after Kinsey, took it up. Jeffrey Weeks has written about how the early gay liberation movement of the 1960s was soon eclipsed by a different emphasis: "'the breakdown of roles, identities, and fixed expectations' [advocated in early liberationists] was replaced by 'the acceptance of homosexuality as a minority experience,' an acceptance that 'deliberately emphasizes the ghettoization of homosexual experience and by implication fails to interrogate the inevitability of heterosexuality'" (Weeks, quoted in Bersani 1987, 203, n.8).

This struggle in the West made homosexuals, and homosexuals made the struggle. That this movement has been successful in many ways (and that it should be welcomed in some respects)[15] should not distract from the fact that it has also made it more difficult to understand erotics. It has helped to reinforce the notion that erotics is the outcome of so-called sexualities.

The struggle for homosexual rights succeeded, after all, not because object choice was different from any of the other sexual fetishes. Rather, it was successful, I would contend, because, after the legalization of abortion and the widespread availability of reliable chemically based birth control in the United States, the trope of biological reproduction no longer culturally singularized and underwrote heterosexual relationships. Why couldn't "homosexuals" enjoy the same (nonreproductive) rights?

But the division of everyone into heterosexuals and homosexuals tended to obscure the other sexual fetishes. Now, it was simply assumed that it is the sex of an object that arouses. But is it? Or is it, say, race, color, wealth, language accent, lower-class style, hair color, smell, being dressed in a leather jacket or a fur coat, masculinity, femininity, penetrating another body, being penetrated, and so on and so on, apparently ad infinitum?

What, then, is a fetish? I use the concept in two ways. The first, made famous by Marx and Freud—what I would call the modernist version—argues that a fetish somehow misrepresents "reality." It attributes a power to something that objectively it does not have. But if we eliminate the assumed teleology of biological reproduction (or socialist revolution), another version of the fetish emerges, one I shall call postmodern: that is, the simple description of social actors' own experience of an attraction that they cannot fully explain, that overpowers and "subjects" an individual otherwise considered "free" and autonomous. Postmodern fetishes just *are*.

The difference between these two versions is often a matter of perspective. The modernist version is typically attributed to others, not to oneself, while the postmodern version invariably rests within the bounds of an actor's own view (which, of course, may be "explained" otherwise by a modernist). I use both, according to context, in this essay.

Science studies theorist Bruno Latour (2010) has recently taken up the concept of the fetish in ways that overlap and differ with my exposition.[16] His concept of antifetishism corresponds exactly with my definition of the modernist fetish, while his notion of the "factish" resembles, in some ways, my version of the postmodern fetish. Where I differ from Latour is the inconsistency with which he rejects modernism. According to him, the modernist fetish must always be a mistake, and in *We Have Never Been Modern* ([1991] 1993), he goes to some length to level the playing field between scientists and others as producers of knowledge. But in *Reassembling the Social* (2005), he takes the diametrically opposed position of arguing, in a classic modernist move, that *his* social theory trumps all others, especially "critical sociology." I believe, in contrast, that contradictory theories can coexist in both the natural and social sciences—in this case, the notions of the modernist and postmodern fetish.

Both Latour's and my expositions are inspired by the remarkable work of William Pietz, who pointed out that all notions of the fetish originated along the coast of Atlantic Africa, in the interaction of European traders and Africans after the fifteenth century. In what follows, I propose to bring a sense of the *longue durée* of Atlantic African history to analyze interactions mediated now by the Internet between African men and gay Europeans.[17]

In the Western metanarrative, men and women in capitalist societies have progressively constructed themselves in terms of "free" wage labor, in opposition to all forms of bound labor—with slavery at the limit. And with regard to political organization, "free" societies are said to require democracy, in which all citizens supposedly participate as equals. Finally, "free" trade and the untrammeled Internet of images and messages have created a density of global interaction that has brought the peoples of the four continents into a new intimacy (Lowe 2015).

However, participating in such freedoms has always required a particular kind of modern personhood—the lack of which has justified social exclusions (Povinelli 2006). Modern persons are assumed to have an interiority in which deliberative reason, rationality, is used to fashion and create the self. So Western liberalism not only exists in relation to an assumed nonmodern outside but also constantly fights an internal battle. As Albert Hirschman (1977) put it, rational "interests" exist in tension with what are assumed to be the "passions" in Western political and economic theory.

What Hirschman did not emphasize is that sex constitutes perhaps the prime passion for Westerners. The notion of the sexual fetish originated precisely in structural opposition to the tamed interests, and in doing so, it became the very epitome of the irrational. Perhaps it is not surprising, then, that the erotic for Westerners has often involved reversals, what we might call the abjection of rationality. In this context, the transgression of law, the assumed primary location of rationality in the West, can become erotic in itself. No more apposite illustration exists than the writings of the Marquis de Sade (carried out, incidentally, during that explosion of supposed reason, the French Revolution). The erotic extends, then, far beyond the question of the sex of an object. But this broader territory has hardly been explored in recent anthropology and history; ironically, nineteenth-century sexology seems to have been much more in touch with this variety—even if a large part of it was interpreted as perversion.

There are a great many quandaries to be faced on this broadened terrain. Perhaps the central one is the difference between power grounded in everyday social life (one might say Marx's or Foucault's kinds of power) and another sort embodied in fantasies and erotic fetishes—as in Freud's and, later, Lacan's exploration of their patients' imagination of the human body, its orifices and appendages, its social openings and closings. These two forms of power may intermesh and reinforce one another but, just as often, *they may not*. Any such connection has to be demonstrated, not simply assumed (and it is mostly assumptions that we have been given so far).

In her clarifying account of recent work on sex and gender, Janet Halley offers the following typology:

> A person framing a conceptual, descriptive, normative, and/or political project that involves a discontinuity between two theories of power, two descriptions of the world, two normative aims, two invoked constituencies, and so on . . . can choose between *converging* and *diverging* them. We could, for instance, decide that normatively it would be terrible to have a theory of homosexuality that was not ultimately feminist, or a feminism that did not wholly encompass our theory of homosexuality; we would then be aiming for complete convergence. Or we could say that it is better for some reason to have some division or autonomy or even conflict between the two projects; we would then be aiming for some degree of divergence. (Halley 2006, 25)

My account is divergentist. There has been a persistent tendency in recent accounts of so-called sex tourism and more widely in some forms of feminism and postcolonialism[18] to take up a convergentist approach that reads fantasies and representations as ipso facto evidence of exploitation. For example, literary critic Joseph Boone (1995, 90), to whom I owe much in this essay, wrote of the "occidental mode of male perception, appropriation, and control." But texts are not lives. Forms of sociality cannot be "read off" texts. In the example I shall analyze below, Atlantic African men reveled in the sexual and racial stereotypes that Europeans brought to their encounters. Europeans' fetishes, in African contexts, put Africans in control.

Many Westerners are disturbed by the very recognition of sexual fetishes (other than their own, of course, which they tend not to recognize as such). Fetishes, after all, transgress the Western notion of love. The desired is seemingly reduced only to a partial and inconsequential part of himself or herself—feet or hair, breasts or penis, age or race. Such partialisms are thought to "other" the beloved. But Freud and Lacan had more complex views of love, and indeed, the power of their theories lies in the ability to make sense of such ambivalence. As I shall argue, the very process of erotization may necessarily involve some "objectification."[19]

Sharon Holland (2012, 46) writes, "I suggest that we can't have our erotic life—a desiring life—without involving ourselves in the messy terrain of racist practice." She poses Emmanuel Levinas's question, "Is the Desire for the Other *(Autrui)* an appetite or a generosity?" (2012, 41). I cannot answer that question for the people I shall describe. It requires a level of knowledge, finally, that I do not have. I would say, though, that the question arises in one cultural tradition (perhaps not all traditions, at least not in the same way) and, within that tradition, it should be raised with respect to all sexual relationships, not just culturally marked, cross-racial ones.

Grounded in history and anthropology (Traub 2013), what follows reflects a wider, interdisciplinary investigation. In some ways, I return to the nineteenth-century sexologists for inspiration. And I hope to show that situations described by literary theorist Mary Louise Pratt (2008) as "contact zones," frontiers in which sexual and other cultural systems come into association, contradiction, and sometimes surprising interdependence, furnish especially rich contexts in which to think the erotic more broadly—my ultimate goal.

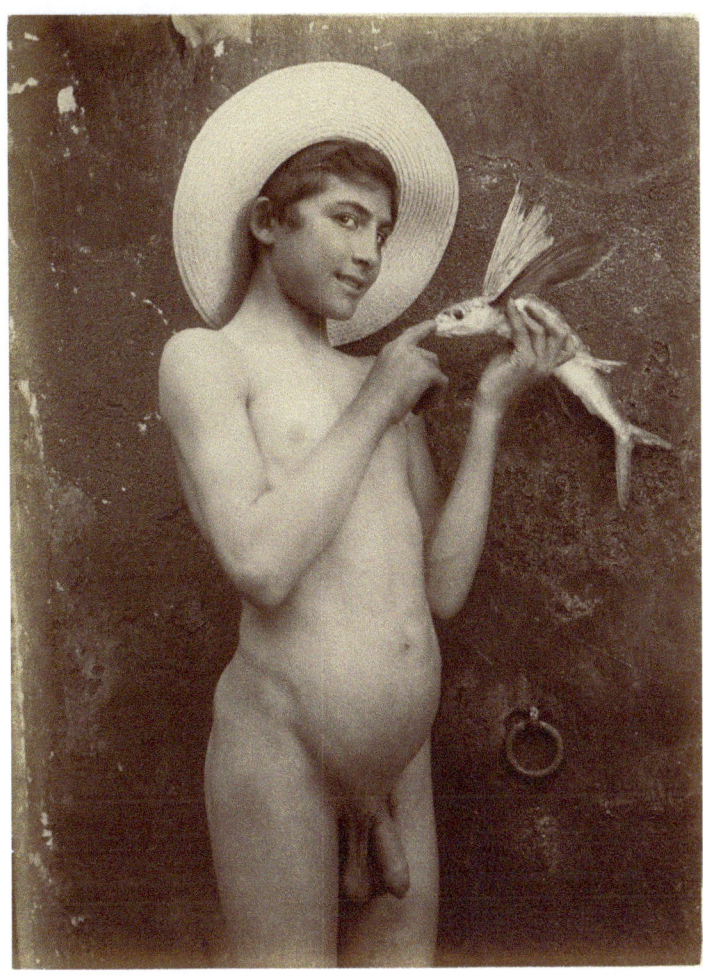

Figure 3. *Ragazzo con pesce volante* (Boy with a Flying Fish), by Baron Wilhelm von Gloeden, c. 1895, courtesy of the J. Paul Getty Museum, Los Angeles.

CHAPTER ONE

Ethnography Interruptus

I first became aware of what I call the contact zone between young Atlantic African men and their European lovers when one of my white gay friends in Oakland, California—"Johnny"—sold his house, located one block from mine, at the nadir of the recent U.S. housing recession, to move to Africa to live with his married-to-a-woman boyfriend. The two had met online.

Johnny's boyfriend, whom I shall call Justice, was a jack-of-all-trades, a bodybuilder in his late thirties, and the son of a prominent local shrine priestess, a practitioner of traditional African religion. Justice spoke English but was illiterate, so he had had to hire a "typist" to chat online. My American friend, in his midforties, was a slender computer wiz, long out as a gay man—with a particular attraction to black men. In current parlance, Johnny had a fetish for black men.[1]

There was not much of a visible gay community in the country to which Johnny moved, one I shall not identify in this book. Colonial sodomy statutes continued to make male-male sex illegal and were occasionally enforced with jail time and (for foreigners) deportation. And local nationalists and Pentecostal Christians increasingly attacked homosexuality as un-African and sinful, as a measure of everything that had gone wrong in recent years. Homosexuality had become a topic for conversation on local radio programs, in newspapers, and in national and international politics.[2] But so far that reaction had not been nearly as extreme as that in Uganda, for example.

As I thought about the sheer improbability of Johnny's coupling, the shock of the present came into focus: it was not only that capitalist media had produced time-space compression of the type analyzed by Marxists like David Harvey (1990). It was also that multiplying and differentiating underground libidinal networks, long localized, had come to the surface and were beginning to connect and interact across the globe (Povinelli and Chauncey 1999).

Neither of these linked transformations, the time-space compression created by capital nor the explosion of differentiating erotic networks, had occurred evenly across space. Because of an ocean-floor cable off the Atlantic African coast and Moore's law that the number of transistors that can be situated on a silicon slice doubles every two years (thereby making computers quickly out-of-date in the capitalist cores but still exportable as secondhand products to the peripheries), the Internet has reached neighborhoods like Justice and Johnny's (for an example, see Burrell 2012). In doing so, it has begun to link people with radically different definitions of the erotic, roles to be taken in sex, and, not least, in love—to dramatically extend and to some degree reterritorialize the "contact zone."

From one point of view, this development has increased the possibilities for love, since the range of possible partners has been so expanded (Baym 2010; Kaufmann 2012). But this very growth has also encouraged a greater specialization of desire. In such a context, sexual fetishes have flourished. Gay Internet sites, for example, sometimes invite participants to list their fetishes—in addition to age, race, body type, and role in sex. But this specialization of desire has also been surrounded by new auras of uncertainty, for Internet "romance scams" and other so-called 419 schemes (a Nigerian phrase from the numbered section of that country's law on fraud) have also blossomed, so much so that U.S. embassies abroad regularly warn of them. After all, the Internet is disembedded from face-to-face channels of communication such as gesture and body language that can confirm (or call into question) truth and sincerity.

As we shall see, the idea of scam—like that of corruption, to which it is related—is defined from a certain (external) point of view. A condemnation from an "outside," the idea of scam can almost always be reenvisioned as an ethical, or at least acceptable, component of the core values of a contrastive "inside." This relativity will become clearer in the presentation of materials to follow.

As soon as I could, I paid a vacation visit to Johnny in his new setting, to discover a working-class urban neighborhood of perhaps four to five thousand in an Atlantic African city, a neighborhood that had started out as something of a traditional village with its own fields far from the city but that had recently been surrounded by expanding, much more expensive suburban housing—villas with high fences and gates. Because the neighborhood, with its much denser settlement, traditional architecture, and open sewers, stood out so clearly from its social surroundings, local inhabitants referred to it in English as the "ghetto."

Inside, relationships between local men and European, North American, and Australian gay men were a kind of open secret.

As many as eight or nine white gay foreigners had, in fact, built second-story rooms above their African lovers' family homes. One German man had built an entirely new three-story home on the urban land of his African lover's family. Before readers assume that these represent recent developments, I should mention Stephanie Newell's (2006) work on a British palm oil trader and writer, whom we would now call gay, in early twentieth-century Nigeria. John Stuart-Young integrated himself into the community by building a second-story room over his Nigerian lover's family house.[3] To sum up, in Johnny and Justice's new neighborhood, anyone could look out over the hillside and "see" same-sex sex—even if they were not supposed to comment publicly upon it.

I found this scene fascinating. At the time, I knew of nothing like it in the African literature.[4] I began to prepare for a year of fieldwork. Back home, I completed the bureaucratic processes necessary for a preliminary project to interview five African men looking for or with foreign white lovers and, if I could find them, five foreigners with or looking for African lovers. I carried out these interviews in August and September 2012.

Strikingly, African men typically represented their European relationships with respect to commodities.[5] If many white gay men came to Africa propelled by the fetishism of race, African men seemed to meet them with what Marx called the fetishism of commodities. One young man was proud to show me, on his cell phone, a picture of himself and his Australian lover, seated on a couch holding hands, in an otherwise unfurnished room, surrounded by unpacked boxes full of household items. His lover had bought them a newly built house in a suburb farther out, but with his lover back in Australia, in the job that paid for all these commodities, and with social life in the new development so limited, the African man often returned to his original neighborhood—where I happened to meet him in a bar.

Photographic images assumed an outsize role for African men. One young man in his early twenties with a German lover in his forties insisted on taking me to his home to show me albums of pictures from a trip to Germany. There was one in which he was decked out in full gear, such as one might see in a gay leather bar in Berlin or San Francisco. Another African man in his late forties had legally partnered with his German lover, an owner of a gay bar in Hamburg, where they both lived and worked for most of the year.[6] The man with the German husband happened to be visiting his wife and grown children in the ghetto while I was there. He kept an automobile in Africa and, as more than one of his neighbors pointed out to me, he had returned to Africa on a German passport. The car and the passport were more than objects. They were icons of success.

Many of the relationships between Africans and foreigners (though not the last one mentioned) had begun in Internet cafés, of which there were many in the ghetto. One or two (before being closed by the police shortly before I arrived) were entirely devoted to young African men educating themselves about Western gay customs, all the way from the difference between tops and bottoms to sadomasochism and master/slave relationships. The principal primer used was gay male pornography, typically viewed while young men also trawled multiple gay Internet dating sites, looking to chat with foreigners. What did Western gay men want? African young men made themselves experts on that question.[7]

Given the local unemployment rate for young men, it was not as if those hours in Internet cafés could necessarily have been spent more productively elsewhere. That time—late into the night, when more foreigners were signed on and when café rates went down—was sometimes devoted to outright scams. After hours of chatting with a lonely older gay man, it was not unusual for the African partner to ask for airfare to visit abroad. I interviewed one older gay man in Oregon who had sent more than $2,000 for this purpose. When the young man disappeared, the man in Oregon felt humiliated because he had known about such schemes, and he still had allowed himself to be used. Two thousand dollars was, of course, a considerable amount in the ghetto and only reinforced the notion that computers could dramatically change lives.

Digital connection, however, produced more than 419 schemes. As we have seen, real relationships and certainly a fair amount of reportedly enthusiastic same-sex sex, in all kinds of combinations and permutations, also took place. Rather than Africans traveling abroad, it was more common for foreign gay men to come to Africa for a visit.[8] Their new African friend usually acted as a tour guide, with the two visiting the usual tourist sites, staying in the same hotels, sleeping in the same bed. Such tours usually covered several countries and nearly always included the rain forest, "the jungle," and, on the Atlantic coast, slave castles, those holding pens that had sent more than twelve million African slaves to the New World. African American tourists experienced the castles as sites for mourning and for reconnecting to their cultural roots (Holsey 2008). Some gay white tourists, I shall suggest, had surprisingly different associations.

Given the link between computers and huge but mysterious rewards, both the Internet and same-sex sex were associated with the occult. Both were transgressions, according to Christians, used to access illicit wealth. It was widely believed, for example, that young men in the neighborhood used charms and spells, provided either by local Koranic scholars *(mallams)* or traditional African shrine priests, to attract foreigners through computers. And it was precisely such evil—pacts with the devil, according to Pentecostal Christians—that were continually denounced in the large and loudspeaker-enhanced churches that ringed the ghetto (denunciations that probably also produced desire).

It was not, of course, only foreign men that were sought. Foreign women were also the object of African attention. One slightly built man in his late forties in the neighborhood confided in me: "You know, this search for a white man is not working out for me. Can you help me find a white woman?" As one young man explained, it was more difficult to attract women on the Internet. Immediate and direct appeals to sex rarely worked (as they did with men). It took more time to reassure, to entice, to romance. Such was more likely to produce results in face-to-face interactions with female tourists to West Africa.

The search for a foreign partner, whether male or female, took place in a setting in which traditional marriage between African men and African women was coming under considerable pressure. Given the unemployment produced by structural adjustment programs, uneducated urban men found it difficult to command the economic resources to support wives and children. Some men in the previous generation had been lucky enough to procure low-paying but secure government jobs. Their sons had been thrown back entirely into the hustle of the informal sector—the very concept of which was invented by Keith Hart (1973, 74) to describe a West African slum: "Nima is notorious for its lack of respectability, for the dominance of a criminal element, and for the provision of those goods and services usually associated with any major city's 'red-light district.' In this environment, the availability of certain illegitimate means (particularly of a casual, rather than a professional kind) is scarcely less than infinite; moreover these activities, while recognized as illegal, and therefore somewhat risky, meet with little of the opprobrium found elsewhere in the city."

Johnny and Justice's neighborhood had some of the same qualities. The 2010s had become even more economically challenging than the 1960s described by Hart.[9] Given that change, a number of men in their late forties in Johnny's neighborhood had never married (and therefore probably never would). They were the local epitome of social failure. They were teased in my presence, and without descendants, they would, for example, never be given showy funerals—the rite that defined, finally, a good life.

It was in this context that male-male relationships with foreigners had begun to subsidize traditional marriage. With increased resources flowing to the African man and his family, the pressures to marry a local woman became irresistible. Even if a foreign gay partner objected, it was not too difficult to conceal a young wife's presence, since, unlike Johnny, most visited for, at most, only a few months out of the year.

After I had returned home from what seemed a remarkably successful three weeks of study, Johnny visited California the following Christmas. I was taken aback to learn that his boyfriend's mother, the shrine priestess, had instructed Johnny that the gods were unhappy with the questions I was asking. Given his commitments to his new family, Johnny said he could not be seen with me again in the neighborhood.

At first, I interpreted the mother's concern as one of protecting local young men—an issue with which I was intensely concerned. But more reflection raised the possibility that the mother wanted to bring me into her orbit and to repair the relationship between the gods and myself (as she had done many times with Johnny).

In any case, I realized that the gods might have a more clearsighted view of the risks involved in this research than the encouraging young men whom I had just interviewed. The latter were remarkably open and candid about the most intimate details of their own and their neighbors' lives. But how much did this forthrightness spring from the hope—no matter how much I explained about academic research and writing a book—that what had brought me to Africa was an attempt to find a lover? So many other white gay men had preceded me that strangers in the street openly flirted with me (a man in his late sixties). They winked and rubbed the palm of my hand with a bent finger when we shook hands.

I thought about what additional ethnographic work would entail. The more I learned, the more local my focus would become, and therefore the more difficult it would be to disguise location. And, of course, there was the local reaction against "homosexuality." I did not want to precipitate a sex panic that would endanger the men who helped me.

I finally decided that what fascinated me was not so much the deepening of ethnographic detail. It was the construction of a theoretical approach that would make sense of such a provocative case—as well as all others I could envision. To my knowledge, no such system existed. In a short period of time, I had collected remarkable materials—so unusual for Africa that I probably would not have believed them without gathering them myself. And Johnny remained a crucial interlocutor, first from afar and then again in California when he temporarily moved back in 2016. After consulting Johnny, I decided I could keep the promises of anonymity to those who had helped me by locating them, only inexactly, in "Atlantic Africa," that narrow strip of the coast from present-day Senegal to Angola that had been in interaction with Europe for over five centuries.

The more I investigated the history of Atlantic Africa, the more I came to realize that it provided, in fact, the keys to my theoretical conundrum. Eventually, I went from Atlantic Africa back to Europe and the United States to question the very notion of sexuality. At its most ambitious, this essay aims to explode Western notions in order to reconstruct the erotic commitments, the fetishes, of social actors across the *longue durée*.

CHAPTER TWO

The Concept of the Fetish

> The term fetishism suits quite well, we think, this type of sexual perversion. The adoration, in these illnesses, for inanimate objects such as night caps or high heels corresponds in every respect to the adoration of the savage or negro for fish bones or shiny pebbles, with the fundamental difference, that in the first case religious adoration is replaced by sexual appetite.
>
> —Alfred Binet, "Le fétichisme"

If what we now term fetishes brought European and African men together in the 2010s, it was hardly for the first time. Atlantic Africa was, in fact, the scene for the creation of the very idea of the fetish.

In a series of remarkable essays, William Pietz (1985, 1987, 1988) laid out an intellectual history of the interaction of Portuguese and then Dutch, English, and other European traders with Atlantic Africans after the fifteenth century. Accounts of European voyages to Africa, such as the one published in 1703 by Dutch merchant Willem Bosman, *A New and Accurate Description of the Coast of Guinea,* found their way into the libraries of some of the most prominent European intellectuals.[1] By the time of the Enlightenment, the idea of the fetish provided Europeans with a potent example of just what reason was *not*—hence Hegel's (in)famous account of the lack of dialectical development in African history.

By the latter half of the nineteenth century, it was becoming clear that the concept of the fetish had little relation to the complexities of West African belief; even so, what Masuzawa (2000) called the ghost of fetishism continued to animate theoretical conversation. Not long afterward, the idea of the fetish had all but died in anthropology, but it had a dramatic rebirth in analyses of Europe itself, after Marx and later the sexologists like Binet, Krafft-Ebing, and Freud imported the idea to describe, respectively, the formation of capitalist economies and European psyches.

For Marx, the fetish of commodities or money—or at the deepest level, capital—involved a misattribution of the power and creativity of human labor to mere things. In capitalism, men and women produce an ever-expanding array of wealth, but ironically, they experience the very things they create as having power over them. Consequently, they bow down and worship the fetish (capital). We say that money makes money and that capital creates.

For Freud, fetishism also involved a displacement from "reality," but the primal story he told involved not the shape of world history but the contours of individual development. The "end pleasure" of reproductive sex (Freud [1925] 2000, 76) could be blocked by an attachment to fetishes—for example, fur or underwear (instead of genitals).[2] The master fetish, it might be thought, would be the father's phallus, but according to Freud, it was actually the mother's. Or more correctly, it was the "disavowal" that the mother lacked a phallus.[3] "Monuments, it was once suggested, are to history as the fetish is to the maternal phallus. In order to deny the absence of something that doesn't exist, you fill the gap, blanking out the absence and endowing this material object [the fetish] with the lineaments of your desire" (Ades 1995, 85).

The fetishistic situation involved, then, a little boy's anxiety that he himself might suffer "castration." Bowing down to a sexual fetish was a way of dealing with the unease,[4] but it was one that could also prevent the boy from finally commanding the power of the phallus and taking his father's place.[5]

Both the sexual scientists and Marx had enormous influence, far beyond intellectuals. Marx's *Capital*, published in 1867 and subsequently translated into many of the world's languages, was one of the nineteenth century's most influential texts, made sacred by early twentieth-century socialist regimes. It set out a historical teleology that promised a final salvation, communism, based not just on liberating individual consciousnesses but on changing the structure of society through social revolution.

Exactly how and when that teleology ceased to be credible to most of the world's population is a story that remains to be plumbed, but certainly after the disintegration of the Soviet Union in 1989, its demise was clear for almost all to see (Buck-Morss 2000; Furet [1995] 1999). The collapse of Marxist teleology was, according to Jean-François Lyotard ([1979] 1984), only one instance of a larger cultural pattern in which all "metanarratives" no longer make sense. In our so-called postmodern age, the allure of commodities became something to be celebrated. Advertisers self-consciously specialized in the propagation of fetishes, and artists like Andy Warhol attempted to capture their magic.

To turn from Marx to the sexologists, Binet is remembered today more for his role in intelligence testing than in relation to theories of sex, but, in fact, he was the first to apply the notion of the fetish to the sexual realm. In his 1887 article, "Le fétichisme dans l'amour," Binet summarized a case described five years earlier by his teacher, Charcot.[6] The case of the eroticized nightcap was then repeated by Krafft-Ebing in his *Psychopathia Sexualis:*

> L., aged thirty-seven, clerk, from tainted family, had his first erection at five years, when he saw his bed-fellow—an aged relative—put on his night-cap. The same thing occurred later, when he saw an old servant put on her night-cap. Later, simply the idea of an old, ugly woman's head, covered with a night-cap, was sufficient to cause an erection. The sight of a cap or of a naked woman or man only made no impression, but the mere touch of a night-cap induced erection, and sometimes even ejaculation. L. was not a masturbator, and had never been sexually active until his thirty-second year, when he married a young girl with whom he had fallen in love. On his marriage-night he remained cold until, from necessity he brought to his aid the memory-picture of an ugly woman's head with a night-cap. Coitus was immediately successful. Thereafter it was always necessary for him to use this means. Since childhood he had been subject to occasional attacks of depression, with tendency to suicide, and now and then to frightful hallucinations at night. When looking out of a window, he became dizzy and anxious. He was a perverse, peculiar, and easily embarrassed man, of bad mental constitution. (Krafft-Ebing [1902] 1965, 175–76)

Krafft-Ebing's work went through seventeen editions from 1886 to 1924, with numerous translations from German into other languages. Freud's *Three Essays on the Theory of Sexuality* subsequently went through six German editions from 1905 to 1925, with even more translations.

Many ordinary readers found in Krafft-Ebing's and Freud's works insights into their deepest selves (Oosterhuis 1997). What had seemed in some cases a vaguely felt but indistinct sense of difference, or in others a deep and lonely secret, came now to be publicly named and described by medical authority.[7] For example, Samuel Steward, growing up in rural Ohio in the 1920s, discovered British sexologist Havelock Ellis's *Sexual Inversion* in his late teen years. According to Steward's biographer, Justin Spring:

> The book immediately set Steward's mind at ease about just who and what he was, and proved a welcome alternative to the vague but terrifying sermons he had heard all through childhood about "sexual sin." Thanks to Ellis, "not only did I discover that I was not insane or alone in a world of heteros—but I also learned many new things to do. I made a secret hiding place for the book under the attic stairs, and read and read and read. Thus I became an expert in the field of sex theory (by the time I finished the book I probably knew more about sex than anyone else in the county) and then began to make practical applications of this vast storehouse of materials." (Spring 2010, 10–11)

Deviations, at least in their most pronounced forms, were diseases according to many early sexologists, but what made sexual fetishes pathologies depended entirely on the assumption that the telos of sex is biological reproduction (see Davidson 1987, 259–62). When that assumption, like other teleologies, no longer made sense to many Europeans and North Americans, the pathology of sexual fetishes began to fall away.[8] The cultural transformation was hardly complete or uncontested, of course, but just the same, it was dramatic. Homosexuality became more or less a benign variation. And even sadomasochism became something of a cultivated art, a kind of postmodern *ars erotica*—at least in certain limited circles in San Francisco and New York, Amsterdam and Berlin.[9]

CHAPTER THREE

African Origins

Let me return to the fifteenth century on the coast of Atlantic Africa. At that point, quite different social worlds came into abrupt collision: on the European side, a late feudal and developing capitalist system of exchange, soon with Enlightenment reason; on the African side, the most baroquely elaborated systems of trade on the continent, with a bewildering multitude of currencies (see especially Guyer 1993, 2004). African traders were animated by cultural projects of self-enlargement in a cosmos in which earthly success always depended on unseen powers and ancestral spirits. The contrast between African and European traders (organized by the Dutch West India Company by the mid-seventeenth century) only increased over time. By Bosman's time, Protestant Dutch traders lived in a natural world evacuated of all spirits.

But how could trade be secured in a space of such fundamental difference? Any formal colonial framework lay centuries away. And Europeans were prevented by African authorities from traveling very far inland. Along the coast, Europeans died of yellow fever and malaria at frightening rates; after a year on the coast, about half were dead. Those who survived did so largely because they took African wives who fed and nursed them through illnesses (Brooks 2003). From the very beginning, then, the contact zone depended upon sexual relationships.

There was already an institutionalized relationship between African "landlords," influential men descended from the first settlers of the land, and African "strangers," or the more lately arrived (Dorjahn and Fyfe 1962). That relationship was easily transposed to Europeans on the coast. "One of the most important privileges accorded resident strangers, European as well as African, was that of consorting with local women—usually women who were related to or dependents of influential persons in the communities who sought to derive additional advantages from affiliations with strangers" (Brooks 2003, 51). It was not long before a racially mixed social strata had developed, though unevenly along the coast (Jones 2013; Jean-Baptiste 2014).

It was precisely in this context in the sixteenth century, Pietz argues, that the modern European notion of the fetish first developed. It appeared in a pidgin term, *fetisso,* derived from the medieval Portuguese word *feitiço* ("magic" or "witchcraft"). Fetissos or fetishes were African religious objects on which European traders were forced to take oaths with their African counterparts to create the equivalent of commercial contracts. It was the fetish that acted as a guarantor; it punished anyone who broke an oath with death and destruction.

> Basically a middleman's word, it *[fetisso]* brought a wide array of African objects and practices under a category that, for all its misrepresentation of cultural facts, enabled the formation of more-or-less noncoercive commercial relations between members of bewilderingly different cultures. Out of this practical discourse

about "Fetissos" and "fatish-oaths," Protestant merchants visiting the coast elaborated a general explanation of African social order as being based on the principles underlying the worship of Fetissos. (Pietz 1987, 23)

> That a fetish was believed to have the power of life and death over an individual was a commonplace of European fetish discourse. This sanctioning power through magical belief and violent emotion was understood to take the place of the rational institutional sanctions that empowered the legal systems of European states (at least those free of "Romish" superstitions). Indeed, the paradox of African society as it was understood in these texts was that social order was dependent on psychological facts rather than political principles. (Pietz 1987, 44)

How did particular fetishes originate? According to European traders, through the chance imprinting by random objects on Atlantic African social actors' projects (Pietz 1987, 43). Bosman reported the following conversation with his main (probably creole) informant about the number of African gods:

> He obliged me with the following Answer, that the Number of their Gods was endless and innumerable. For (said he) any of us being resolved to undertake any thing of importance, we first of all search out a God to prosper our designed Undertaking; and going out of Doors with this design, take the first Creature that presents itself to our Eyes, whether Dog, Cat, or the most contemptible Animal in the World, for our God; or perhaps instead of that any inanimate that falls in our way, whether a Stone, a piece of Wood or any Thing else of the same Nature. (Bosman 1703, quoted in Pietz 1987, 43)

Clearly, such descriptions related more to European obsessions than to the cultural projects of African actors.

What, then, from an African point of view, were the objects that Europeans called fetishes? The most developed answer in relation to Pietz's work has been offered by Wyatt MacGaffey (1977, 1988, 1990, 1994) in relation to the *minkisi* (singular, *nkisi*) of the Kongo (see also Blier 1995; Blier formulates her analysis solely in terms of local African concepts, in this case across what used to be called the Slave Coast). The word *nkisi* could be used to refer to a spirit, an amulet, a statue, a medical treatment, or a living priest.

In relation to the objects Europeans called fetishes, *minkisi* were spirits of the dead who had been made to take up residence in a "container" like a bag or a calabash or a carved statue. These latter did not "symbolize" spirits. Rather, they were spirits' containers—when properly composed by a priest with the requisite knowledge. If profaned, spirits could leave, in which case objects became "empty," mere objects.

Properly composed, *minkisi* acted in the world of the living: they healed diseases, brought the rain or banished it, punished thieves, killed witches, and confirmed agreements. In this way, according to MacGaffey (1988, 203), "the dead, revitalized through the human properties attributed to the objective foci of ritual, replaced the living in taking responsibility for affliction, accusation and punishment."

In contrast to these African ideas, the European concept of the fetish, to sum up Pietz's analysis, was of an object of "untranscended materiality." That is, it was an object that did not refer to anything outside itself but was assumed (falsely, from the European perspective) to behave like a person. Fetishes had personalities.

Particular fetishes originated in radically singular, random events that brought together otherwise heterogeneous elements. The power of the fetish thereafter rested upon its enduring capacity to fix and to repeat these coincidences. Such "fixations" involved the bodies of living men and women—with the fetish

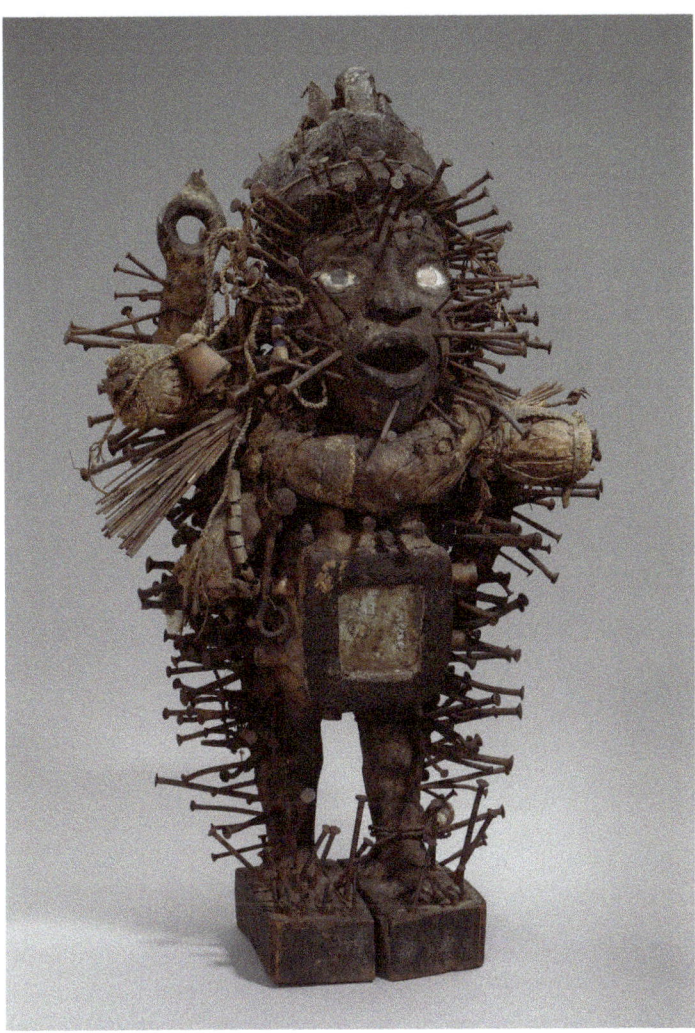

Figure 4. A Kongo *nkisi*, unknown carver, early twentieth century, courtesy of the Minneapolis Institute of Art, The Christina N. and Swan J. Turnblad Memorial Fund. Shelton (1995, 220) speculated that Kongo *minkisi* may have represented Christian influence: representations of Christ nailed to the cross "provided powerful images, with sado-masochistic overtones which clearly articulated suffering and bodily denial as a path to eternal life and the attainment of supernatural authority."

being a kind of "external controlling organ" of their bodies, affecting and effecting their life, health, and fortune.

For centuries, these elements of the European notion of the fetish were encased in a fundamentally critical point of view. "The discourse of the fetish has always been a critical discourse about the false objective values of a culture from which the speaker is personally distanced" (Pietz 1985, 14). But this critical aspect—what made fetishes inferior and misleading forms of reasoning—was abrogated when Western teleologies (like the inevitable expansion of reason) no longer commanded respect. In the present, fetishes are simply the mysterious and ineffable ways that individuals experience the specifics of erotic arousal or the attractions of commodities.

Ironically, however, much of their Atlantic African origin remains: to the extent that fetishes can be cognized, they continue to be traced to chance fixations, usually during childhood. Consider the following richly contextualized case study in 1980 by Gosselin and Wilson—in which the subject has clearly, if only indirectly, been influenced by the deep history I have recounted. Chance associations continue to fix fetishes:

> Mr. W. is now forty-five years old. He was born of reasonably well-to-do parents, but his father died when Mr. W. was three years old and his mother went to live with her brother at a seaside resort ... He became passionately interested in natural history, an interest that has persisted all his life, and states that his first memory of rubber, the fetish material that now dominates his sexual life, was the smell and feel of a hooded jacket and overalls made of rubber-backed cotton that he wore during some of his walks in the country in search of wildlife. "In such a situation," he says, "one is alone, undistracted by any stimulus coming in and highly sensitized to everything. Under these circumstances it seems to me inevitable that I should have begun to turn on to something,

especially something which proclaimed itself, by smell and noise and the heating effect upon my body, like that rubber did. The odd point about it is that I don't remember it at the time having anything to do with sex." It was in fact not until the age of fourteen that Mr. W. had what he describes as "the sort of experience that you psychologist fellows dream about." He had, he says, returned from a country walk, dressed in his water proof outfit. He called out to see if his mother was at home. At first, she didn't answer him, but after a while she came downstairs and greeted him. After a while, the uncle appeared as well: "And although nothing was said, I somehow was convinced that they had been having sex together." [Mr. W. was happily married but kept his fetish a secret. After fifteen years of marriage, his wife died.] He made no serious attempt to acquire another partner, because he was "pretty much able to look after himself" and the appearance of his house bore this out. His fetish collection grew speedily after his wife's death, and until recently—for he is at present working on a job overseas—he kept in his house a complete "rubber room" lined throughout with curtains of the same material and containing two large cupboards full of rubber garments, gas masks, photographic and other equipment. He has in the past visited specialist prostitutes to play out some aspect of his fantasies, but now does not do so, feeling that he has all he needs for sexual satisfaction without leaving home. (Gosselin and Wilson 1980, 49–51)

Following Max Weber's work on religion, we might say that Mr. W. had become a virtuoso of the fetish.

Over the twentieth century, what was fetishized—the result of what appeared as the most personal and individual of tastes—was yet a part of wider social transformations (Gosselin and Wilson 1980, 47). Nightcaps, with their smell of hair and associations with the night, seem to have disappeared. Body parts like feet, hands, hair, breasts, and butt remained, but as touching became perhaps less tabooed, did the frequency of such fetishes decrease? No longer do we hear, for example, of men who cut and steal girls' hair on the streets. Sexy underwear and rubber, vinyl, and leather outerwear make their first appearances.

Various kinds of uniforms constituted fetishes in the early twentieth-century European underworlds described by Magnus Hirschfeld. Soldiers were the principal object of attraction, and the minutiae of military insignia were finely appreciated.

> Within every group there are always very strong differentiations. For example, among the "wooers of soldiers," we find ones who tend toward men's organizations, and among them also those who "fly" almost exclusively to noncommissioned officers, while others almost always prefer orderlies. Then, there are ones who occupy themselves only with officers. Besides this, the different types of troops play a role. For many, only the infantry exists, for others the cavalry, for a third the marines. I know a homosexual for whom only the "First Ulan Guards" were of erotic significance; it seemed the rest of the German army did not exist for him. (Hirschfeld [1920] 2000, 336)

And the fetishization of the military took place against a wider field:

> Many male prostitutes take a lot of trouble to keep certain fetishistic peculiarities of taste in mind. For this reason, many wore high boots with spurs or sports outfits, sweaters, scarves hung loosely around their neck, jockey or peaked cap; even small lockets or small leather straps in a buttonhole really prove to be effective fetishes. In Berlin, Paris, and London it is no different; you can find walking the streets sailors, who have never been on a ship, jockeys who have never mounted a horse, chauffeurs who have never driven a car, and soldiers who have never held a weapon. (Hirschfeld [1920] 2000, 823)

And, finally, Hirschfeld reports the presence of antifetishes, fetishes that turned off sexual arousal.

C, a former Catholic priest, in his early forties, reports the following. He recently met a young tradesman who in every respect, in his appearance and nature, had corresponded to the type he made into the object of his attraction. They formed a deep mutual friendship. C used to meet his friend after work and accompany him home, which gave him more pleasure than he ever experienced. One evening both went to the circus. Afterward the younger man accompanied C home. Here, for the first time, C hugged him and said all kinds of flattering things about his handsome appearance. The tradesman replied rather naively, "Well you should see me next Sunday in my new suit and my yellow shoes!" At the very instant C heard the words "yellow shoes," all his excitement disappeared. He was unable to touch the young man. He could not at all understand the change in his nature. He could hardly shake his hand when it soon became time to say goodbye. The cooling off accompanied by a sentiment of strong antipathy can be explained by C's feeling an aversion to yellow shoes that he himself did not comprehend. He could hardly even speak to people who wore such shoes. He had also even attacked a pair of yellow shoes. While he was on vacation and staying at a hotel, in the early hours of the morning he crept out of his room and in the corridor found a pair of yellow shoes that had been left out. He tore them to shreds with a pocket knife. (Hirschfeld [1920] 2000, 355)

We can recognize a certain continuity between Hirschfeld's cases and the present. For example, Chicago-based Samuel Steward (he would later move to Oakland), born in 1909, obsessively kept a sex diary of all his encounters, and by the 1970s, he would estimate that of the 807 men with whom he had had sex, a significant proportion was servicemen: "sailors—a coupla hundred; sergeants—about 30; marines—2 dozen" (Spring 2010, 85).

But an obsession with the military clearly declined over time, in the United States at least. As I shall explain later, when urban communities of gay men devoted to masculinity first developed in the 1950s, they took their style from motorcycle gangs, with leather jackets and chaps—not so much from the military. And by the 1960s, the time of gay liberation, the United States was, of course, involved in a highly unpopular war in Vietnam. The counterculture began to emphasize a certain male androgyny.

In sum, each fetish appears to have a social history of its own—a topic about which we so far know relatively little.

CHAPTER FOUR

The Poverty of Sexuality

> The current conceptualization of homosexuality as a condition is a false one ... It is interesting to notice that homosexuals themselves welcome and support the notion that homosexuality is a condition. For just as the rigid categorization deters people from drifting into deviancy, so it appears to foreclose on the possibility of drifting back into normality and thus removes the element of anxious choice.
>
> —Mary McIntosh, "The Homosexual Role"

One of the first questions that European gay men asked themselves in Johnny and Justice's neighborhood was something like "Is this African man *really* gay"? On Internet sites and in person, Africans presented themselves as "gay," but as we have seen, other aspects of their lives seemed (to Europeans) to stand in contradiction with this claim. In all, it was not my impression that African men were much concerned with the question of sexuality.

It is fairly common, as I have already pointed out, in sexual cultures across the world for those who penetrate in male-male sex to be thought of as ordinary men. Unlike today, when our current notions of homosexuality mark *both* partners to a same-sex act as deviating from the norm, as little as a century ago, things were different across many areas of the world: only men who were penetrated, orally or anally, were marked as "queer."

Did some similar conceptual sorting, on the part of Africans, facilitate the meeting of gay Europeans and Africans in the ghetto? The answer appears to be no. While most Europeans in Johnny's neighborhood were apparently (mostly) bottoms, this was not universally the case. One German man was said to be a total top. Moreover, two European "bottoms" reported to me that at some point in their relationships, their African lover had asked if they wanted to switch roles (and one had). The sexual versatility of African men seems to have made the question of whether they were *really* gay beside the point—for their European lovers. One said, "If my friend had been born in Europe, I'm sure he would have been gay. Straight men just don't do what he does."[1]

My information on the intimacies of same-sex sex between Atlantic Africans and Europeans is strikingly paralleled by the account by Nii Ajen (apparently a pseudonym), an African author in Murray and Roscoe's (1998, 133–34) pioneering volume. Let me quote at some length:

> Three white European gay males I interviewed who live in West Africa with their boyfriends spoke of their mixed feelings because of their lover's marriage and partial commitment to their relationship. All three of them admitted enjoying sex profoundly with their African men and only wished they could have had them for themselves alone. Interestingly, the three lovers they spoke of were all said to be extremely versatile in their erotic behavior with their male partners and also in their social roles.

A survey I conducted in London during 1994 of fifteen men born and raised in West Africa who moved to Europe no later than 1990 and who have sex with men regularly provided the following information. They were between the ages of twenty-three and forty. Of the fifteen, four were exclusively homosexual, the other eleven saying they don't mind sleeping with a woman. What was more striking was that two of the eleven said they have problems with sleeping with women, yet cannot think of living without a woman in their life. Also, only two of the fifteen accepted the label "gay." Both were effeminate, exclusively homosexual, and exclusively receptive (that is, "bottoms"). The other thirteen refused the label outright, as they see "gay" as a Western, stigmatized label... Thirteen of the fifteen also had childhood sexual experiences with friends or schoolmates before puberty. Three of them were anally raped as children. The other ten learned from friends, schoolmates, or caregivers. Eleven are versatile in their sexual roles now. The other two discovered sex long after puberty: one at age twenty-two and the other at age twenty-five. The two who had their first experiences in their twenties said they were exclusively insertive ("tops"). Although they admitted to enjoying same-sex intimacy whenever they have it, these two indicated that they do have moments when they feel bad about going to bed with men.

So what was the "sexuality" of these African men?

It is useful, at this point, to compare sexuality to ethnicity. There are, of course, disagreements among scholars who study ethnicity, but virtually no one would now argue that ethnic "essences" propel behavior. In certain contexts, people can be mobilized under an ethnic banner to carry out various goals, all the way from the formation of communities, to campaigns for liberal rights, to violence and the elimination of others (Donham 2011). In this way, "ethnicity" provides identity terms that can be taken up by actors themselves, attributed to others in certain contexts, and even embedded in bureaucratic state structures. But whatever ethnicity is, it is hardly an essence or a state of being—except to its true believers (and then even they inevitably fail to enact purity).

If a social actor claimed, for example, that he had no choice in some matter, that his deep sense of ethnic identity (say, Zuluness) compelled him toward a certain act, few observers would take this as an adequate explanation. Yet a great many do with respect to sexuality. The inadequacy of doing so is, I take it, the central point of historian Joan Scott's discussion of individual experience as historical evidence: "We need to attend to the historical processes that, through discourse, position subjects and produce their experiences. Experience in this definition then becomes not the origin of our explanation, not the authoritative (because seen or felt) evidence that grounds what is known, but rather that which we seek to explain, that about which knowledge is produced. To think about experience in this way is to historicize it as well as to historicize the identities it produces" (1991, 779–80).

So what if any kind of sex, like any kind of culture, is a potentiality for anyone? What if sex is learned, what if it reflects not only cultural definitions, as the social constructionists have argued now for decades, but also, crucially, subgroup social pressures (see especially Reiss 1961)? The position I am advocating emerges in one of Silvan Tomkins's brilliantly detached discussions of how bodily drives can be consummated:

> The drive system has a limited degree of substitutability of consummatory objects. Quite apart from the restrictions of appetite of food, liquid, and sex objects, which are learned, hunger can be satisfied only by a restricted set of organic substances, thirst by a restricted set of liquids. Sexuality has a greater freedom of possible satisfiers since almost any object which is not too coarse in

texture might be an adequate stimulus for stimulating the genitals, although the number of maximally satisfying possibilities is much more limited. The need for air is perhaps the most restricted in terms of the number of possible substitute gases. (Tomkins 1995, 59)

The erotic, what turns people on, is not only constituted, then, in relation to the zones, appendages, and orifices of the body that Freud so insightfully mapped and that Tomkins analyzes above but also, in turn, is activated and ultimately given meaning by wider social and historical transformations, in contextually variable ways.

To advance this argument, let me return to the last half of the nineteenth century. According to Arnold Davidson (1987), following Foucault ([1976] 1978), it was only then that the notion of sexuality was created. It did not exist before. And it was formed in the discourses of the sexologists we have already discussed. In sum, sexuality was and continues to be an assumed organization of individual psyches that produces (or is deflected from) reproductive sex. Types of perversions—homosexuality, fetishism, and sadomasochism—constitute their own distinctive forms, defined always by their structural opposition to reproductive heterosexuality.

The notion that every individual "has" a sexuality has grown more and more ingrained in European and North American thought.[2] This notion can be seen in how titles of iconic works on sex have been translated into English. For example, the German title of Freud's famous work, first published in 1905, that we know now as *Three Essays on the Theory of Sexuality* was *Drei Abhandlungen zur Sexualtheorie,* or, as it was in fact first translated, *Three Contributions to Sexual Theory.*

The adjective, "sexual," continually modifies and therefore moves, but the noun, "sexuality," denotes a determinate state of being with distinct predicates. The seemingly innocent transformation of an adjective into a noun tends to obscure, then, what Davidson specified as the genius of Freud in relation to the other sexual scientists, namely his blurring of the boundary between the normal and the abnormal. In perhaps the most famous footnote of the *Three Essays,* Freud ([1925] 2000, n. 11) wrote: "Psycho-analytic research is most decidedly opposed to any attempt at separating off homosexuals from the rest of mankind as a group of a special character. By studying sexual excitations other than those that are manifestly displayed, it has found that all human beings are capable of making a homosexual object-choice and have in fact made one in their unconscious."

Today, Foucault's *The History of Sexuality, Vol. 1,* has eclipsed Freud's text for many, but the irony of Foucault's title is apparently often lost (Jordan 2015). The grandiloquence of the title should have been the tip-off. The French subtitle, *La volonté de savoir* (The Will to Know), was dropped from the English translation and replaced by the anodyne *An Introduction,* but the French phrase captures Foucault's arguments more accurately. Indeed, the argument of Foucault's book is precisely to deconstruct the notion of sexuality, to show that it is an effect of the discourse created by the sexologists' will to know rather than any actually preexisting psychic, much less biological, condition.

Irony of ironies, then, that the sexual scientists' categories eventually got adopted, in what Foucault calls a "reverse discourse," by so-called deviants themselves. This is Foucault's doubly ironic account of "the history of sexuality" in the West. Given his enormous influence at present, it is altogether surprising to see his supposed followers pluralizing "sexuality" into "sexualities"—as an assumed progressive, more inclusive theoretical move.

I want to emphasize an implication of Foucault's argument that he himself did not explicitly draw out:[3] that there must have been more same-sex sex *before* the notion of homosexuality than afterward. It is, of course, almost impossible to present data to back up such a claim. But Rocke's (1996, 5) study of records from Renaissance Florence is provocative: "In the later fifteenth century, the majority of local males at least once during their lifetimes were officially incriminated for engaging in homosexual relations."

And then there is the "naturally occurring experiment" of prisons in the United States. Regina Kunzel (2008) argues that straight prisoners indeed found erotic pleasure and even love with other men.[4] She shows how the discourse on violent prison rape beginning in the 1960s acted as a kind of screen against recognizing the deeply emotional bonds that existed between some men. Well into the twentieth century, prisons were organized by the opposition between "jockers" (who were straight) and "punks" (who were queer). But in practice, this opposition was continuously undermined. "San Quentin inmate and novelist Edward Bunker cited a 'jocular credo' that 'after one year behind walls it was permissible to kiss a kid or queen. After five years it was okay to jerk them off . . . After ten years, "making tortillas" or "flip-flopping" was acceptable, and after twenty years anything was fine'" (Kunzel 2008, 185).

African men in the ghetto made these transitions rather more quickly. Or, more accurately, we might say that they faced no such "transition" in the first place.[5]

CHAPTER FIVE

African Sexual Extraversion and Getting into Bed with Robert Mapplethorpe

If the erotic spreads over social life much farther than the telos of reproduction would suggest, how do we come to grips with this situation? Georges Bataille provides, I believe, a beginning:

> Eroticism, it may be said, is assenting to life up to the point of death. Strictly speaking, this is not a definition, but I think the formula gives the meaning of eroticism better than any other. If a precise definition were called for, the starting-point would certainly have to be sexual reproductive activity, of which eroticism is a special form. Sexual reproductive activity is common to sexual animals and men, but only men appear to have turned their sexual activity into erotic activity. Eroticism, unlike simple sexual activity, is a psychological quest independent of the natural goal: reproduction and the desire for children. (Bataille [1957] 1986, 11)

Bataille notices that all human societies, as opposed to animal ones, set taboos around two areas of life—sex and death. Sex is typically carried out in private. And we dispose of the dead. Our closest animal relatives do neither. These two observations are linked by Bataille. The erotic is a kind of death, a dissolution of personhood, a glimpse into the most fundamental religious experience of continuity. And the taboos around the erotic are not merely negative ones. "We can," Bataille writes, "even go as far as the absurd proposition: The taboo is there in order to be violated" (64).

From erotics, Bataille quickly jumps to some of the most fundamental aspects of religious experience, opining along the way, "In one sense, the Christian religion is possibly the least religious of them all [because of its relative anti-eroticism]" (32). We need not follow Bataille to all his positions to appreciate two points: (1) the erotic is not defined by the telos of reproduction, and (2) transgressions of sexual taboos are built into the very structure of the erotic. Unstable, the erotic changes over time. Forms of human sociality depend upon the erotic, and as forms of sociality vary, so do erotics.

With this framing in place, let me turn to Atlantic African forms of sociality. For some time, one of the most insightful theorists of African politics has been Jean-François Bayart ([1989] 1993, 2000). He has argued that African forms of relating rest upon patterns of what he calls "extraversion." Social actors, rather than deepening exploitation of their own dependents, build power by pursuing relationships of external dependence— all the while using the cunning and guile of the prototypical trickster in West African folktales to turn apparent subordination into power, at least locally.

Some scholars have questioned the explanatory weight that Bayart attempts to place on this syndrome. And to an anthropologist like me, having first done fieldwork in East and South Africa, it seems to capture a pattern perhaps not continental, but particularly *West* African. Indeed, one wonders whether this orientation to the social world was not some adaptation to the upset and upheaval caused by the Atlantic slave trade. However that may be, "extraversion" is a striking idea that unifies much disparate work, from studies of so-called scams to the novels of Francis Nyamnjoh (2011). And in the present context, it uncannily captures the case at hand: young Atlantic African men on gay Internet dating sites looking for European lovers. What was their "sexual orientation" (Ahmed 2006)? We might answer, after Bayart: extraversion.

West African vodun carvings appear to provide an usually striking illustration of this argument. According to Suzanne Blier's African interlocutors, the statue's penis is associated with trickery. "The penis is associated with Legba, a deity of trickery, communication with the gods and sexual potency. Erect phalluses distinguish this latter deity's shrines and ritual objects" (1995, 147–48). Power and potency, sexual and otherwise, depend upon communication and sometimes trickery.

It should be clear by now that the neighborhood my friend had landed in was quite different from its surrounding cultural context. Inside the ghetto, African relationships with gay Europeans were more or less approved. This was not easy in some cases and certainly not public. But such relationships enabled a kind of continuity in Bataille's terms; I discovered that African male-European male sexual relationships had existed at least as far back as the fathers of the young men I interviewed and probably farther. Before the Internet, men in the ghetto had placed personal ads in European and North American gay publications by mail in the 1980s. As little as a decade earlier (Meeker 2006), any number of changes in communicative infrastructure—for example, what the post office would accept as mail—had laid the necessary groundwork for how sexual minorities would make contact. Atlantic African men from the ghetto were soon "linked in," even before the Internet would once again transform sexual connectivities.

One father and son worked in tandem to entice Europeans. Another young man I ran into was named for his father's European lover: Angus (to change the name but to keep its Scots flavor). One particularly successful man of around fifty, who had a computer and a modem at home, and who had had a German lover when he was younger, offered himself as a go-between for the young men of the neighborhood. "They are all my kids," he said. He offered advice and guidance about European gays, the unstated assumption being that he would receive gifts from the boys when the latter received monies from their new friends. Same-sex sex was a communal project in the ghetto, one that was subject to competition and jealousy as well as help and sharing of information. It was not uncommon for young men to attempt to take away the European lovers of their neighbors.

African wives sometimes protested. One apparently stood outside her house and shouted to the neighbors, "You know what my husband is doing in there? He's fucking that white man." But the neighbors quickly sat her down and asked her just how she thought that she and her children were being supported. She needed to respect that or go back to her parents. This kind of social pressure created an ambiguous and fluid social situation in which one's self could be expanded to the degree that he (usually but not always males) could manipulate the hold of fetishes over others.

If African men's erotic inclinations were focused on extraversion, what about the white Europeans, North Americans, and Australians who found their way to the ghetto? What was their "sexual orientation"?

One German gay man I interviewed said, "I am attracted to black men. Not only that," he said with a laugh, "my black friends tell me I'm attracted to *ugly* black men." An Australian man pointed out that there were very few black men in his country. He had had an aboriginal boyfriend early on, but the last four of his boyfriends had all been African, all from the ghetto. From what I could tell, most of the white men in the ghetto had a fetish for black men. "I can't explain it," one said. "There is just something about the texture of black skin."

As I have pointed out, racial fetishes remain controversial, especially to racial minorities in North America. Racial fetishes often focus precisely on those physical aspects targeted by racists themselves: what Fanon called "epidermalization" being perhaps the central one. But no African I interviewed in the ghetto interpreted white attractions as racism. Just the opposite—Africans seemed pleased to celebrate such attractions, which, after all, represented something of a reversal of typical colonial patterns. One recounted his white lover's delight and surprise when the lover first saw his penis. In addition, many Africans interpreted white enthrallments as the result of the power of the ritual charms they had procured. In other words, white attractions to blacks were typically read as a confirmation of African power.

If anyone were exploiting anyone—and this is not the idiom I would choose in this situation—Africans, it was my impression, typically enjoyed the upper hand, in Africa. That they themselves viewed the situation in this light would seem to be corroborated by the fact that they treated Europeans as "wives" (as I shall explain in the conclusion). That is not to say, of course, that Europeans did not enjoy more "power" in some global sense. They had white skin and passports and relative wealth. They could go home—but, of course, their fetishes kept pulling them back to Africa.

That pull was, it is clear, embedded, even if with a different valence, in some of the same phantasms as white racism. Not long after the earliest years of European expansion, a white-is-just-right story proved remarkably enduring over the centuries, one that linked race globally with gender. To simplify (racism is already a simplification, of course), Africans, both male and female, were thought to have too much body and not enough mind. Consequently, both African men and African women were *masculinized* in relation to whites. That made African men supermales and African women incompletely feminine, compared to whites. Conversely, Asians were thought to have too much mind and not enough body. Both male and female Asians were *feminized* in relation to whites. That made Asian men incompletely masculine but Asian women superfemales.[1]

This Lévi-Straussian pattern of oppositions created African males and Asian females as spectacular figures of libidinal interest. As early as the seventeenth century, European travelers began commenting on the sexual equipment of African men, their "large Propagators" (Hyam 1990, 204). And Asian women became the symmetrical opposite: refined, submissive, and beguilingly beautiful Madam Butterflies, the subject of Italian operas.

Writing of the eighteenth century, Bleys (1995, 90) contends: "The Enlightenment debate on other races' natural status ... was very clearly marked by an ascription of sexual qualities. This was shown perhaps most prominently in the ascription of 'feminine' characteristics to the people of America, Asia and the Pacific, while Sub-Saharan Africans and Arabs were most commonly accredited with a rather exaggerated and 'uncivilized' masculinity."

The point of whiteness was that it was "just right," not unlike the story of the three bears' porridge—too hot, too cold, just right. In other words, the structure of racism is not always a simple hierarchy with whites "on top" (Paul n.d.). It can represent a more complex notion of proper balance.

The sexual attractions to African males and Asian females that arose out of these investments were not symmetrical, of course. To be attracted to an African man was potentially to participate in the fantasy of being overpowered, whereas being attracted to an Asian female was potentially related to domination itself.

The irony of these racial fantasies, in relation to black men in the United States and Europe, is that in reality, few had any real power at all. They were themselves abjected in a system of racial capitalism. So how did white racial fetishes form? Almost no research has been done on this question, past Mumford (1997) on the North American example of the 1920s. My speculation, following Bataille's discussion of transgression, is that black men become intensely erotic figures (for some white men and women) when they appear to reverse and challenge the actual system of racial domination.

Photographs of black bodies accomplishing such reversals (such as, say, the famous black power salute from the 1968 Olympics) may have played a role in creating racial fetishes. Before the pervasiveness of photographic images, the imprinting of fetishes upon social actors depended upon unmediated seeing (sometimes complemented by the more evolutionary ancient senses of smell and touch). Afterward, the camera not only conveyed fetishes but also may have played a role in propagating them.[2] Such a focus on the mediation of sexual fixations is not new. Lawrence Stone (1992) proposed that flagellation was first spread to the middle classes in England when engraved pornography became widely available in the early eighteenth century.

Compared to etching, photography has perhaps an elective affinity with race in that it can capture skin tones so subtly.

Whether these speculations have any value, by the end of the 1970s, racial fetishes were common in North American gay communities. Black men attracted to white men were known as "snow queens," white men attracted to black men, "dinge queens." White men attracted to Asians were called "rice queens," Asians attracted to whites, "potato queens." By the 1980s, bars and social organizations based on these fetishes existed in most gay communities in the United States (see M. Smith 1983). It was not unusual for the interracial organizations based on these attractions to take the lead in attacking the evident racism of the gay community itself.

For the quintessential example of a white man with a fetish for black men, let me turn to Robert Mapplethorpe. His photograph *Man in Polyester Suit* is often called his masterpiece, a designation that works in more than one sense. When he first confronted it, the black gay critic Kobena Mercer attacked the photograph as racist, as did others. Later he significantly modulated his position. I would suggest that the photograph be read as a depiction not of black men per se but of white fascinations with them, Mapplethorpe's in particular (Morrisroe 1995, 234).

According to Luc Sante (1995, 47), Mapplethorpe's photographs "do not show sex as much as they enact it, locating the act in the exchange between the photographer and whoever looks at his work. The viewer is pressed into service as proxy partner, top and bottom at once. The reactions of Jesse Helms and his ilk would no doubt have given Mapplethorpe satisfaction—their horror only proves that he succeeded in getting them into bed with him."

Man in Polyester Suit is, of course, focused on the black phallus. The punctum of the photograph, in Roland Barthes's terms, is the engorged and uncircumsized black member with a slight glistening at the tip.[4] The work is, in its entirety, devoted to the contrast between the luminosity of the black skin and the flatness of the polyester suit, an industrially produced material not unlike other fetishized materials like rubber or vinyl.

It is easy to be reductionistic about the black phallus. Take the case of Johnny. There were, after all, many black gay men in Oakland. He hardly needed to go to Africa to find one. There was clearly something else, some supplement that drew white gay men to the African ghetto. This was, I believe, the difference that Africa offered by the beginning of the twenty-first century. The heady days of black liberation in the United States—and of the Black Panthers, closer to Johnny's previous home in Oakland—were decisively over. Africa furnished another frontier. And postcolonial Africa, compared to the United States, was no longer structured by racial domination, even if white privilege remained (Pierre 2013). That meant that white men's fetishes for black men did not so immediately raise the recall, as it did in the United States, of blacks' quotidian experiences of white racism.

In a sense, white gay men in Johnny's new home were something like anthropologists of an earlier day (see Grinker 2000 for the example of Colin Turnbull). They were attracted by cultural difference. They were attentive to structures of world power that marginalized Africans. And they often took up local projects that resembled those of activist development agents— setting up libraries for local children, microfinancing for local small enterprises, and so-called appropriate technology transfers. In some real sense, it was the overdetermined "meaningfulness" of this situation that kept whites coming back. Africa provided a kind of stakes for living that was missing at home, even if most whites only visited for a few months out of the year.

CHAPTER SIX

Para-ethnography, Golf, and the Internet

How did ordinary, nonelite Africans in Johnny's neighborhood learn enough to "trick" with European gay men? I'm using "trick" here both in the gay sense of having sex with and the African sense of outwitting. I have already suggested the most recent part of the answer: the Internet. Indeed, sexual extraversion and the Internet were in many ways preadapted to one another. First of all, as often has been pointed out, the Internet expands the role of fantasy and possible deception. But, secondly, the Internet dramatically increases the possibilities for gaining cultural knowledge about others. The need for such knowledge is particularly great when the intent is to some degree to deceive ("con men have to be smart") and when the others in question are themselves members of an evolved and sometimes subterranean subculture.

In a felicitous phrase, Douglas Holms and George Marcus (2008) recently called the process of interpretation of cultural others on the part of everyday actors "para-ethnography." Anthropologists, then, are not the only ethnographers. This being so, anthropology as an endeavor can become a kind of ethnography of ethnographers in some situations. For social actors, action in the world increasingly takes place with an awareness of—indeed a cultural theory of—alternate cultural worlds.

The Internet hardly created para-ethnography in Atlantic Africa, but without doubt, it has recently expanded its reach and depth. As we have seen, centuries ago, the contact zone introduced other cultural worlds to Atlantic Africans—eventually in dramatically violent ways. The colonial administrations that resulted, at least in the Gold Coast (Ray 2015), began to attack the centuries-old relationships between European men and local women, not so much because of the mixed-race children they produced (who were absorbed into the African population), but because of the leverage that African "in-laws" had traditionally exercised over European "husbands." With African women off limits, and many fewer European women in the colonies than men, the colonial order began to create significantly homosocial spaces.

It would surely be a mistake to call colonialism a gay project, but colonies attracted northern European white men drawn to other men (T. E. Lawrence, Roger Casement, and E. M. Forster being perhaps the most famous). But para-ethnography in colonial contexts, at least for illiterate Africans, was highly delimited and almost entirely sustained by forms of face-to-face communication. For ordinary Africans, these took place in domestic spaces in which houseboys, cooks, and gardeners came into sustained contact with white men and sometimes white women (Stoler 2010). And—critical to the case at hand—certain kinds of sports, like golf, offered yet another venue.

Golf as we know it seems to have begun in fifteenth-century Scotland, where it was played in the roughs along the seashore.

At times, Scottish kings tried to suppress the game since, unlike archery; it held no military value for the state. By the nineteenth century, golf was an elite avocation in Great Britain and had spread to British trade depots and colonies.

The secret of the uniqueness of Johnny's neighborhood is, I believe, its location next to a colonial-era golf course. Let me consider what a cultural innovation in landscape a golf course instituted. Before, chiefs had given Africans access to land in order to plant their swidden fields and to graze their animals. African landscapes reflected the residue of these layered processes (which to Europeans always seemed visibly disordered). When the golf course was established in the 1930s, a fence was built around the perimeter, enclosing an area into which ordinary Africans could no longer go, much less graze their animals. Foreign species of trees were planted. Holes were laid out, and the grass was mowed. To Africans, this space must have "summarized" colonialism: a powerful white fantasy they could not understand and from which they were excluded.

But Johnny and Justice's village was to some degree the exception. European golfers required caddies, after all, and young boys from Johnny's neighborhood quickly took up this role. Indeed, they organized to keep out other boys, situated just a little farther away. Personalized relationships between older European golfers and young African caddies developed in which African boys left their school lessons when "their" Europeans showed up at the tee. By the time of colonial independence, boys from the ghetto had worked as caddies for Europeans for more than three decades—against a regional history on the Atlantic African coast that extended much farther back. In the eighteenth century, British slave traders had built a two-hole golf course on Bunce Island, where they were "served by

African caddies dressed in kilts especially woven in Glasgow" (R. Shaw 2002, 29).

For decades before the end of colonialism, then, boys from the village that became the ghetto accumulated and shared knowledge of white culture. It is perhaps no surprise that a few of the relationships between golfers and caddies turned sexual. I gathered stories of two instances, one from a man in his twenties, another from one approximately fifty. The latter recounted, with evident great pleasure, stories of a European flight steward in the 1970s who blew a horn that played his airline's radio advertising jingle as a signal that he had arrived at the golf course. Hearing the jingle, the African young man knew to come to the course. The two not only played golf over the time of the steward's layover. They ate and drank and had sex in the steward's hotel room. Through support from the steward, the African young man eventually made his way to London, where he lived for a number of years, in relationships with British gay men. Through these experiences, he gained a kind of worldliness that was altogether unusual for men of his background. In 2012, after his Belgian lover had died, he continued to live in Johnny's neighborhood during the week but visited his wife and children on the weekends in a nicer neighborhood not far away.

We can now begin to appreciate, I think, why fucking a white man had become erotic for some African men. The answer has little to do with our notions of sexuality. Fucking, I take it, is always associated with feelings of power. After colonialism, when African men penetrated white bodies, they also imaginatively reversed colonial interdictions that had excluded them from wider cosmopolitan worlds. And to the extent there was some ruse involved, the humor that resulted must have added to the pleasure. What I am suggesting is that the wider terrain of desire *always* slides into and inflects the erotic. At some point, these two realms become impossible to separate. In her study of black women and the pleasures of racialized pornography, Jennifer Nash (2014a, 452) writes, "My understanding of pleasure is capacious—it is an understanding that includes, of course, erotic and sexual pleasure, but that also includes political pleasures, humorous pleasures, pleasures in transgressing, pleasures in making use of and then upending racial fictions."

Golf prepared the way for the Internet. Both golf and the Internet provided the same kind of window onto a wider, desirable world. As so-called romance scams, both straight and gay, became notorious in Atlantic Africa by the 2000s, many North American and European websites blocked posters with IP addresses from the region. But at least one European gay site did not, and it became the site of choice in Johnny's new neighborhood. On a more or less representative day at 11:00 A.M. California time in 2014, almost 100,000 Europeans were signed on to the site—with about 30,000 Asians, 800 North Americans, 1,000 Middle Easterners, and 1,700 Africans.

Given their peculiar postcolonial history, the men in Johnny and Justice's neighborhood knew how to appeal to European gay men. Stories about sex with European men had circulated for decades in the ghetto before the Internet arrived. When cheap secondhand computers in Internet cafes began to make their inroads, strikingly, a few men posted photographs that depicted themselves almost exactly as Mapplethorpe had portrayed his African American lover—faceless and focused on their penis. The website asked its posters to classify their own penis size as S, M, L, or XL. About 80 percent of Africans said they were XL. The wider gay pornographic obsession with penis size to which Africans were responding was apparently fairly recent, according to Waugh (1996, 324). It seems to have appeared only after the 1930s, after the invention of portable cameras and close-up lenses.

Profiles coupled two basic themes: African sexual superiority along with the desire for a long-term relationship, ideally marriage. Some profiles were quite short. "Dreaming to Be with You and Marry if Possible." "Really hope to find the right man in my life to spend the rest of my life with." "I am looking for a soulmate, the one who will care, love me and satisfy me." One had perhaps copied an African American Internet profile: "im a cuul cutie out here looking for relationship n shit im very down to earth n very cuul to hang out wif gooogle me niggas if yall wanna noe more."

Some were humorous: "I'm the male reproductive part of the flower." "Hi there. I am a hard master here seeking a slave to train hard who will pay every two weeks." "Am looking for an old man who is ready to meet me for a serious relationship." "I want you to get swept away. I want you to levitate. I want you to sing with rapture, dance like a dervish, because we give hot and crazy sex and hot fuck. Have you experienced sex in the jungle before?"

One young man presented himself as a master for European slaves in a particularly historically inventive way. In his profile, he pointed out that during colonial wars, when European soldiers were taken captive and held by African forces, they were raped. They were raped so expertly that the Europeans began to appreciate it. This illustrates, the profile claimed, why and how Africans make the best masters—a dramatic reversal, of course, of the actual realities of colonial conquest.

CHAPTER SEVEN

White Slavery

I am thirty-five years old, mentally and physically normal. Among all my relatives, in the direct as well as in the lateral line, I know of no case of mental disorder. My father, who at my birth was thirty years old, as far as I know had a preference for voluptuous, large women. Even in my early childhood, I loved to revel in ideas about the absolute mastery of one man over others. The thought of slavery had something exciting in it for me, alike whether from the standpoint of master or servant. That one man could possess, sell or whip another, caused me intense excitement, and in reading *Uncle Tom's Cabin* (which I read at about the beginning of puberty) I had erections. Particularly exciting for me was the thought of a man being hitched to a wagon in which another man sat with a whip, driving and whipping him.

—Richard von Krafft-Ebing, *Psychopathia Sexualis*

In spring 2004 [after the photographs of torture at Abu Ghraib were circulated], I read a scene report—a written description of a consensual BDSM play scene—in the Janus newsletter. The scene took place at a San Francisco dungeon in late March 2004. It was

> an interrogation scene, involving a colonel, a captain, a general, and a spy. The spy was hooded, duct-taped to a chair, and slapped in the face. As she resisted, the spy was threatened with physical and sexual violence, stripped naked, cut with glass shards, vaginally penetrated with a condom-sheathed hammer handle, force-fed water, shocked with a cattle prod, and anally penetrated with a flashlight. The scene ended when the spy screamed out her safeword [the signal that the scene was no longer consensual] "Fucking Rumsfeld!"
>
> —Margot Weiss, *Techniques of Pleasure*

When I sent Johnny a first draft of this essay in 2015, he wrote back to say that he thought I had not properly understood the role of SM in the social scene I was describing. While I had interviewed one African man who had in fact related his role in SM scenarios with white visitors, Johnny was correct: I had placed the man under the rubric of the computer scams in which he was involved rather than in relation to SM.[1]

As my relationship with Johnny deepened, it emerged that he himself had been seriously involved in SM, as early as his college days. As time went on, however, he felt increasingly alienated from the SM scene in the United States. It had somehow lost its "authenticity," he said. Indeed, his travels to Atlantic Africa were, in some ways, a response to that perceived loss.

In addition to our numerous conversations, Johnny sent me four photographs that he had copied from the profile of an African master posted to the European gay website I have already described. He assumed that the photographs had come from the neighborhood in which he lived or nearby. These images, more than any of Johnny's words, even those that described the most intimate of details, transformed my understanding. All four photographs involved the same African master with the same white slave. The face of the master, a heavyset black man of maybe thirty-five, was clearly visible in some of the shots, but the face of his gray-haired and balding white slave, perhaps in his fifties, was obscured.

Had the slave requested the photographs as a memento of his visit? And then the master discovered his own purposes for the pictures? Or had it been the other way around? Or was it some collaboration from the very beginning, a part of the erotics of the interaction? Clearly the photographs had taken some preparation to produce. The slave was naked except for a basic tunic such as one might see in a movie about Roman slaves. The locales were rural, either in thick forest or in a distinctly African field. The master wore his street clothes.

One image in particular held my attention. The white slave, sketched in Figure 5 overleaf, head down, facing the viewer, was wielding a traditional African hoe in a rural field, chained to his African master, who was "driving" him with a whip from behind. And observing from the other side of the picture were two skinny boys, in their late teens perhaps. This image captured, at the same time, an act that was erotic, clearly for the slave and perhaps for the master; an image that could be used to recall that arousal and reproduce it, both for the original participants and for others; and finally, a kind of local classroom on white erotics.

The photographs sent me to the literature on SM. The ethnography of what is now broadly called BDSM in the West, bondage-domination-sadism-masochism, has just begun. It holds unusual challenges. I have found sociologist Staci Newmahr's ethnography, *Playing on the Edge*, of a pansexual SM scene in a large northeastern American city particularly insightful.

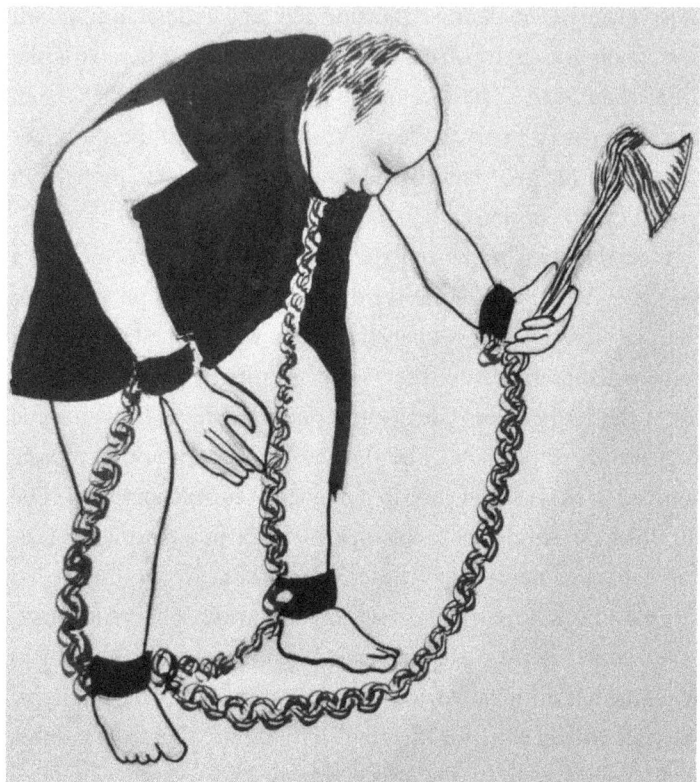

Figure 5. A sketch of the central figure of a white slave from a photograph attached to an African Internet profile. Not shown (to the left and behind) are the African slave driver and (to the right and behind) two African boys observing the scene.

Her reflections on her own bodily sensations during and after SM scenes were revelatory. Newmahr (2011, 18) defines SM as "the collection of activities that involve the mutually consensual and conscious use, among two or more people, of pain, power, perceptions about power, or any combination thereof, for psychological, emotional, or sensory pleasure." She insists that SM is neither simply an alternative sexual practice, for everyone, nor role play, for everyone (2011, 60).

Rather, she puts dominance/submission at one pole of SM and pure "pain play" at the other. D/s clearly depends upon role play and is typically highly eroticized. Pain play, on the other hand, according to Newmahr, can be independent of both role play and sexual arousal. Whether the value of these distinctions will be confirmed by further research, I do not know. It is noteworthy, however, that Newmahr's distinctions more or less mirror those of Tomkins, of which Newmahr seems to have been unaware:

> Sexual sadism consists in the conjoint heightening of anger, excitement, and joy, as well as sexual pleasure. Sexual masochism is the mirror image of such a complex, in which one ordinarily identifies with the role of *both* victim and victimizer. There is usually, though not necessarily, a collusion between sadomasochistic partners such that double identification is shared at the same time that each also plays a distinctive complementary role. They need each other to share the total scene *and* to play distinctive roles of angry aggressor who inflicts pain and victim who suffers pain. Humiliation and degradation may, in addition, be conjoined with pain and suffering. If so, the sadist is excited by his disgust and or contempt of the self and of the to-be-degraded other, and the masochist is excited by the identification with the contempt of the other and by the experience of being hurt, disgusted, humiliated, and degraded. Some sadomasochistic sexual relationships may magnify humiliation primarily rather than the infliction of pain, with or without anger. The texture of sadomasochistic sexuality varies therefore with the ratios of anger and humiliation, excitement and enjoyment, and sexual pleasure versus inflicted pain. (Tomkins 1995, 202)

For my purposes, both of these authors are useful in introducing African SM, which appears to me more focused on the erotics of dominance and submission than on the infliction of pain.

That African SM exists at all is, of course, something of a surprise. I know of no prior report of its existence. After all, slavery as a social institution remains a touchy topic in much of present-day Atlantic Africa. As Kopytoff and Miers (1977) explained in a classic analysis, African slavery, unlike New World varieties, typically incorporated slaves into local lineages and kin groups—over varying lengths of time and with different degrees of lingering stigma. To refer to matters of slave descent in the present, particularly in public, reflects, at the very least, bad manners (Holsey 2008). In this context, the foreignness of Europeans and their obliviousness to such concerns seem to have allowed a different approach to "slavery."

Also striking is the seeming open-mindedness of Africans. This occurs at a time when most gay Europeans and North Americans themselves, not to mention others, continue to view SM as "weird," if not "sick." The development of lesbian SM communities in the United States in the 1970s, for example, produced an enormous backlash from some feminists (see Rubin 2011). And as late as 1987 in Great Britain, a case of consensual SM was legally prosecuted as assault. Likewise, in the United States, "In 2000, a police raid of a private party in Attleboro, Massachusetts, resulted in arrests on assault changes, despite the fact that no alleged victims pressed charges" (Newmahr 2011, 7).

Why was the African reaction to SM different? It was, I believe, the very nature of extraversion that allowed Africans to contemplate sexual practices quite unlike their own with little apparent disgust or shame (often the reaction, after all, to others' fetishes). The point was to use their relationships with powerful outsiders to accomplish internal cultural goals. To accomplish this, Africans turned themselves into pure ethnographers, learning how to apprehend the world from an external point of view, one uncontaminated by their own moralisms (which continued, of course, to be applied in other contexts).

From the other side of the relationship, why were Europeans drawn to Africa as a site for SM? One can construct various beginnings for SM. Anthropologist Paul Gebbard (1976, 165–66) pointed out that sadomasochistic practices seem to occur only in highly stratified societies with developed forms of symbolic mediation like literacy. As words, sadism and masochism were coined by Krafft-Ebing at the end of the nineteenth century—after the novels of the Marquis de Sade and Leopold von Sacher-Masoch had made their marks. And Freud ([1925] 2000, 25) noted what he believed was the composite character of sadomasochism (an argument disputed, for example, by Deleuze): "The most remarkable feature of this perversion is that its active and passive forms are habitually found to occur together in the same individual. A person who feels pleasure in producing pain in someone else in a sexual relationship is also capable of enjoying as pleasure any pain which he may himself derive from sexual relations."

For Western gay men, the story begins after World War II in the development of what began to be called leathersex.[2] Not all men in leather communities were devoted to SM, but SM defined perhaps its core. At that point, the overwhelmingly dominant definition of a male homosexual focused on his supposed effeminacy, and indeed gay men themselves, as shown by Esther Newton (1972) in her brilliant analysis of drag queens, not infrequently cultivated flamboyantly effeminate styles.

By the mid-1950s, an emerging network of gay men in New York and Los Angeles began to reject this way of being gay and to adopt hypermasculine styles.[3] This development was institutionalized in so-called "leather communities," in which masculine men sought out other masculine men, networks united by a certain rebellious form of brotherhood that was socially focused in urban bars and motorcycle clubs.

Hard, black shiny leather—whether in motorcycle jackets, caps, tight-fitting chaps and pants, or heavy workman's boots—became the defining fetishes.[4] And for a core of the men—though not for all—SM and other forms of kinky sex became a deeply meaningful part of their lives. By the 1970s, this new erotic constellation of gay masculinity, leather fetishism, and hard-core SM had spread not only to other American cities like San Francisco and Chicago but also abroad to Sydney and London, Amsterdam and Berlin. It is perhaps not surprising that leathermen's quest for the masculine eventually led some to black men—who, as we have seen, had long been masculinized by the Western semiotics of race.[5]

Consider perhaps the most famous gay SM novel ever published, *Mr. Benson*, written by John Preston for serialization in *Drummer Magazine* in the late 1970s. The back cover blurb of the 1983 edition summarizes the plot: "Jamie wears his tightest jeans to the leather bar and makes sure the handsome, unsmiling top across the room gets a good view of his assets. But this is no ordinary leatherman, no weekend daddy: this is Mr. Aristotle Benson. Lucky Jamie is about to get an education and to begin his journey from a cute but forgettable clone to a compliant, hard-bodied slave, sensitive to his Master's every glance and gesture."

Mr. Benson, a wealthy white New York master, shares his slaves with other masters—two black masters in particular, Tom and Brendan. The latter is a policeman who lives in Harlem with a white slave named Rocco. Below, Jamie, the slave protagonist of the novel, talks with Rocco:

I was desperate to compare notes. "What's it like, Rocco?"

"It's hell, just hell. Sometimes he'll bring home that other guy Tom." I nodded to show him I knew who Tom was. "Well, they'll break into the house and they'll start this game thing that they're living in that period. I have to figure out what it is and who I'm supposed to be. It's always something racial. Like last week they came in and they were making like we were in Africa and that I was a white slaver they had captured. They were supposed to be tribal chiefs. Brendan put on this real heavy, real primitive music. And they were wearing African clothes. They used my body to make up for all the African children that had ever been sold off to America as slaves.

"And another time Brendan brought by these four other cops. They were all black and all had dicks that could kill you. They make believe I was a dope pusher who was selling heroin in the ghetto and ruining the lives of black teenagers. They took their revenge by gang-banging me, one after another, till each one had fucked me at least twice. I was bleeding for days.

"He's always pulling things like that, Jamie. Every night when we listen to the news, if there's anything on the tube that tells about a white person doing something to a black person, I get it—I get fucked, or he ties me up and goes to find people to work me over, or he'll take me to a back room bar where I have to suck off every single black person there." (Preston 1983, 81–82)

Tongue-in-cheek complaint, this fantasy illustrates how the actual history of power can condition, through reversal and redefinition, the constitution of the erotic.

A similar structure of feeling is recorded in the sex diary of white Samuel Steward, a tattoo artist in Oakland, California, in the late 1950s: "Most of all at present . . . I enjoy [the black bodybuilder] Bill Payson . . . It is his attitude of semi-cruelty, you might say, that I like; not cruelty exactly, but more a feeling of 'This is what you deserve, white boy, you scorn me because I'm a nigger, and here I am... that'll show you what I think of you'" (Spring 2010, 246).

Biman Basu argues that it was the consumption of nineteenth-century slave narratives from the American South that, through reversal, structured many twentieth-century European SM scenarios. The original impulse for the creation of slave narratives was, of course, quite different. Henry Louis Gates Jr. has shown how it was the very act of writing that was being used to illustrate the modern personhood of slaves, their interiority and rationality, just like whites. Therein lay the moral monstrosity of slavery. But once abstracted into symbolic discourse, signifiers could float. They could be transformed and reversed to serve other, imaginative uses.

> In addition to the devices, instruments, and methods [of punishment of Southern slaves], certain episodes are repeated in both the slave narratives and in sadomasochistic narratives. One such episode is having a slave whipped by another. Both masters and mistresses sometimes employed others to administer corporal punishment. When a "gentleman wishes his servants whipped, he can send him to the jail and have it done..." If she does not wield the whip herself, a mistress has a slave whipped when the slave "displeased her"... "Many mistresses will insist," after having a slave flogged, on the slave's "begging pardon for her fault on her knees, and thanking her for the correction." (Basu 2012, 39–40)

Unlike gay romance, the advent of SM in Johnny's neighborhood seems to have depended entirely on the coming of the Internet. Now, Africans had access to voluminous materials on the intricacies of the semiotics of SM, and they could demonstrate, through easily reproduced photographs, their own command of its theater.

Africans advertised as both slaves and masters on the Internet. Did masters learn their trade by first being slaves? Slaves in their Internet profiles invariably recounted the discipline of past masters: "This boy has experience as a BDSM slave to four Masters so far. Sir, it is strong, muscular and available to serve all of Master's needs. It can serve you while you travel here, visit you at home for a trial, or stay forever if you wish to keep it forever." Such presentations of self demonstrated some insider knowledge of SM conventions (but probably not much real experience). *Master* is capitalized, *slave* is not. A slave is referred to as *it*. And a master is addressed as *Sir*.

Given the history of the Atlantic slave trade, one might think that what Europeans devoted to SM were after in Africa was verisimilitude, the added frisson of having a *black* slave. And indeed this may have appealed to a few. But ironically—or perhaps not—it was far more common for Europeans to come to Africa looking for a master, not a slave.

And African masters, in response, typically presented themselves in their Internet profiles as the zenith of animal-like, racialized masculine power—in a remarkable reading of just what white slaves wanted:[6] "A jail that is a dominion of sexual darkness where you will be condemned to be made the humiliated helpless victim in the orgy of naked mass rape that takes place every night, where you will be hanged on your wrists and tied up on your back with widened thighs or simply get dragged to the ground or to my bed where hundreds of those hot black animals spread your legs and make sodomy-sex . . ." The grammatical mistakes—whether intended or not—probably heightened this master's "authenticity" to European and North American readers.

That a much greater demand for masters than slaves exists in leather communities is a recurrent joke. Tom Magister (quoted in Thompson 1991, 91) only half-seriously wrote: "The general consensus in the Leather Community is that there are about ten slaves for every Master. If you factor in the men who switch roles from Master to slave and back again, the ratio gets higher. As for men who are exclusively Masters, they are a fondly remembered breed."

Magister was playfully exaggerating, presenting himself as the last of a dying breed, the top who never bottomed. So when the more earnest sociologist G. W. Levi Kamel addressed the same question, he wrote, "Leathermen themselves agree that participants prefer the passive role by approximately three to one" (T. Weinberg and Kamel 1983, 173). Some African men undoubtedly were "switches." But there can be no doubt about which role was in greater demand in Africa or which held the greater reward.

I was able to interview one African master, a rather unattractive man in his late thirties with something of a potbelly. Unlike others, he presented himself as little interested in romance. "I'm a scammer," he said. He was involved in various forms of Internet schemes, some involving credit card numbers. The scam he carried out on gay Internet sites involved the promise of a live sex show via his videocam. He insisted that anyone interested had to provide payment up front. After collecting money at the local Western Union, he typically never signed on to his computer at the designated time. But once or twice he actually carried through on this scheme and hired two younger, more attractive men from the neighborhood to perform sex online. When the men's families found out, they took the scammer to a traditional form of dispute settlement and demanded that he pay restitution—which he did.

I had asked to speak to the man because I was interested in scammers. But in the middle of the interview, unbidden, he recounted how he had been visited by a slave from Germany. He had played the master, keeping the man caged in his house during the day and having rough sex at night. As he told the story, his face lit up for the first time. It was clear that he had thoroughly enjoyed himself.

I conducted this interview, like others, in an outdoor café in the middle of the afternoon, when few other patrons were around. At some point, I typically offered to buy my interlocutor a drink. Some chose a soft drink. Some preferred beer. Before I could offer, the scammer called the waiter over and ordered the most expensive meal on the menu—for which I ended up paying. I was reluctant to protest since I had felt an I'm-going-to-take-advantage-of-you undercurrent throughout the interview. In many ways, scamming seems to have provided perfect training for being a master: the ability to convey, as an actor might, a feeling to an audience—in this case, a sense of threat, an unconcerned, masculine coldness.

CHAPTER EIGHT

Love and Money, Romance and Scam

> Desire describes a state of attachment to something or someone, and the cloud of possibility that is generated by the gap between an object's specificity and the needs and promises projected onto it. This gap produces a number of further convolutions. Desire visits you as an impact from the outside, and yet, inducing an encounter with your affects, makes you feel as though it comes from within you; this means that your objects are not objective, but things and scenes that you have invested attachment-value in, in a way that converts them into objects that prop up your world. So what seems objective and autonomous in them is partly what your desire has created and therefore is mirage, a shaky anchor. Your style of addressing those objects gives shape to the drama with which they allow you to reencounter yourself. By contrast, love is the embracing dream in which desire is reciprocated: rather than being isolating, love provides an image of an expanded self, the normative version of which is the two-as-one intimacy of the couple form.
>
> —Lauren Berlant, "Desire"

Mutual enjoyment is possible, for example, if you enjoy body contact and I enjoy body contact. A somewhat different type of mutual enjoyment may involve body contact but also the wish to cling to the other. The embrace is capable of being experienced as mutually rewarding if each clings to the other. The embrace also provides mutual enjoyment when each wishes to hug the other, or to hug and be hugged simultaneously, to achieve a claustral interpenetration in which each is inside the other. If each wishes to rub the skin of the other and to be stimulated in the same way at the same time, a particular type of embrace will satisfy both individuals. If each party wishes to take into his mouth, to suck or bite, some part of the body of the other, mutual enjoyment is possible so long as each does not object to the same behavior on his own body. It is possible if you enjoy looking at me and I enjoy looking at you. It is possible if you enjoy looking at me and at the same time my looking at you, and I enjoy looking at you and at the same time your looking at me; in short, our looking into each other's eyes. Mutual enjoyment on a looking basis may, as in the latter case, involve mutual awareness of what each is doing at the same time or, as in the former case, it need not involve mutual awareness. We may enjoy each others' company in the latter case with each looking at the other but without doing this simultaneously and without awareness of mutuality. Thus two people may be quite companionable each involved in reading a book and from time to time one raises his eyes and looks and smiles at the other without the other's awareness, and conversely. Adolescent loving is not infrequently carried on at a distance, with each party stealing glances at the other.

—Silvan Tomkins, *Shame and Its Sisters*

Gay romance, as I have said, was much longer established than SM in Johnny and Justice's neighborhood. By the 2000s, the typical pattern began with several months, sometimes longer, of Internet chatting, after which the white gay man visited Atlantic Africa as a tourist.

In that moment, two very different cultural constructions of love and money began to come into collision. And whether the wealthier and otherwise more powerful white gay man realized it or not, the balance of power tilted decisively toward his African partner. For the white man was stepping back in European time, as it were, to a social world in which homosexuality was illegal and in which blackmail and extortion were always potentialities. After any misunderstanding, it was easy for an African lover to go to the police to claim that he had been molested by a gay foreigner. The police arrested the foreigner and extorted bribes, which were shared with the young African man.

Such recourse was often understood by the African lover as just punishment for a European's taking advantage of him. According to both African and European interlocutors, young men in the ghetto were quite jealous of one another. They were ready to undermine the European relationship of another. And if their own lover did not come through with showy support, they could feel humiliated in relation to their peers. However this sense of self in relation to others eventually worked out, it was not as if Africans necessarily began with the intent to scam. Most, I would say, genuinely wanted a relationship—even if they had little idea of what such entailed from a European point of view.

Misunderstandings were built into this situation. As we have seen, the Europeans who came to Africa looking for a male sexual partner always identified as gay. But sex, for many, was something that could be enjoyed in and of itself, outside of any further social commitment. The same men had, of course, notions of "love," but love is defined as something deeper and more long-standing than sexual attraction, and it was typically opposed to strictly economic transactions. "Love is what money can't buy." If money intervenes too overtly in a relationship, prostitution is the category that comes to denominate it—not love.

According to my research, African men looking for a European partner brought different notions to their encounters. Though many presented themselves as "gay" on European gay social networking sites (a handful listed themselves as "bisexual"), none, as far as I can tell, understood themselves as exclusively attracted to men. Sex with a man was erotic, but that hardly meant that sex with a woman was not. Second, virtually no sex took place between an African and a European that did not involve the flow of economic resources, not as "payment," but more globally as that which constituted the relationship (Cole and Thomas 2009). "No romance without finance," as the African saying goes in relation to men and women.

Not only that, but money and the vision of escape abroad apparently also effected sexual arousal. One young informant (who claimed to have no sexual experience with men—only a kiss) said, "Desire is all in the mind. Someone may get really turned on when he is having sex just by thinking of all the things that will come his way." Almost everyone I talked to claimed that any man in the neighborhood could have male-male sex with a European. But, tellingly, more than half of my interlocutors claimed that they were turned off by the idea of sex with an African man. On the European side, I talked to one man who said that his African partner had virtually raped him on their first date. "But I couldn't believe it," he went on to say. "In the middle of all this hot sex, the guy turned over in bed, relaxed on the pillow, and asked me whether I could buy him a taxi!"

If money turned sex on, its lack could turn it off. Like African wives, male partners to Europeans could go on "sex strikes." They withheld sex to get what they wanted. One stopped having sex with his European partner because the latter refused to buy him another house in a better-off suburb. He wanted out of the ghetto, particularly for the future of his children. The European man, in contrast, enjoyed the difference and vitality of the ghetto.

The clash of cultural perspectives, in effect, set up a kind of filtering process for visiting Europeans. Many left disgusted. A few posted racist reactions on the profiles of those whom they believed had used them. Others ended up paying bribes to escape. But the ones who survived to establish long-term relationships had to take up para-ethnography themselves. They had to develop some appreciation of the different cultural situation in which they were operating. They also had to be generous. One European who had been visiting for years apparently ran up significant credit card debt at home in order to fund his friends in Atlantic Africa—debt he was able to pay off only when his mother died and he inherited. Another invested in a local business with his African partner to the tune of several hundred thousand dollars.

Conclusion

Toward an Understanding of Erotics

It is looking more and more as if the model of (homo) sexuality with which I grew up, and whose genealogy I have tried to map... never had more than a narrowly circumscribed reach. That model never succeeded for very long in establishing a concept or a practice of sexuality wholly defined by sexual object-choice (same sex or different sex) to the exclusion of considerations of gender identity, gender presentation, gender performance, sexual role, and social difference. It never completely decoupled sexuality from matters of gender conformity or gender deviance, from questions of masculinity and femininity, activity or passivity, dominance and submission, from issues of age, social class, status, wealth, race, ethnicity, or nationality. And canons of homosexuality and heterosexuality in their turn installed their own norms of gender identity and sexual role, while seeming to insist with breathtaking categorical simplicity on the "sameness" or "difference" of the sexes of the sexual partners. It turns out that such notions of sameness or difference contained their own hidden stipulations about the condition under which members of the same sex could really be considered the "same," or had to be classed, despite the sameness of their sexes, as actually "different."

—David Halperin, *How to Do the History of Homosexuality*

In this eight-minute short, a museum guard, a middle-aged man of African descent played by Thomas Baptiste and referred to in the credits only as the Attendant, has a sexual encounter with a white man played by John Wilson, called the Visitor. Their attraction to one another takes place in relation to F. A. Biard's 1855 abolitionist painting "Slaves on the West Coast of Africa" which is displayed in the museum. This painting, the film's first image, shows a slave market. There, a white, presumably European man straddles a prone, presumably African man, as other black and white men look on or continue their business. In the periphery of this scene, more white men whip, bind, inspect, and brand other black men. During an ordinary day on the job, the Attendant meets the seductive gaze of the Visitor, and the Biard painting suddenly and literally comes alive. It metamorphoses into a tableau vivant of an interracial sexual orgy, with the participants posed exactly as they were on the canvas, only now wearing modern SM gear. After the museum finally closes, the Attendant and the Visitor consummate their lust by whipping one another in a room off the main gallery—or the Attendant may simply imagine this happening, the film leaves this ambiguous.

—Elizabeth Freeman, on Isaac Julien's short film *The Attendant*

What makes sex sexy? To begin to answer that question, I have suggested that the concept of the fetish provides an essential beginning—an idea that originated, as we have seen, in the contact zone of Atlantic Africa, centuries ago. Tastes beyond rationality, attractions that operate like external controlling organs of the postmodern body, fetishes are contextual and can coexist, sometimes in contradictory ways, and they can change, sometimes dramatically, more often in a person's younger years, but occasionally later as well. And—perhaps most importantly, as in SM—fetishes can be cultivated as tastes can be "educated." They depend upon an infrastructure of mediation, social interaction, and historical context.

The discourse on the fetish is a part of a much larger conversation in social theory about how persons and things interact, an exchange that includes, besides Marx and Freud, Marcel Mauss's famous account of the gift, and into the present, Bruno Latour's (2005, 2010) formulations of actor network theory. All of these approaches problematize, in different ways, the assumed boundaries of persons and things, or persons and parts of persons treated like things. These processes, in the present case, created passions so strong that they propelled bodies halfway around the globe, altering the material contexts of other bodies in ways perhaps impossible to imagine otherwise.[1]

Here, sexual fetishes became parts of scripts for fantasies that aroused bodies to sexual excitement. According to John Gagnon and William Simon's pioneering 1973 book *Sexual Conduct,* such scripts occur on at least three levels: that of the internal psychic reality of an individual, in scripts for social interaction between two or more individuals, and finally with respect to cultural scenarios that recur across social contexts. After the Internet, sexual actors have explicitly labeled their intrapsychic fantasies as "fetishes," inviting others to participate in social interaction, typically drawing on wider cultural narratives.

In 1979, psychoanalyst Robert Stoller began his book *Sexual Excitement* with the following playfully tedious paragraph:

> It has surprised me recently to find almost no professional literature discussing why a person becomes sexually excited. There are, of course, innumerable studies that have to do with that tantalizingly vague word "sexuality": studies on the biology of reproduction, masculinity and femininity, gender roles, exotic beliefs, mythology, sexuality in the arts, legal issues, civil rights, definitions, diagnoses, aberrations, psychodynamics, changing treatment techniques, contraception, abortion, life-styles, transsexual operations, free-ranging and experimental animal behavior, *motoro*, pornography, shifts in age of menarche and loss of virginity, masturbatory rates, research methodology, bride prices, exogamy, incest in monkeys and man, transducers, seducers, couvade, genetics, endocrinology, existentialism, and religion. Statistical studies of the external genitals, foreplay, afterplay, accompanying activity, duration, size, speed, distance, metric weight, and nautical miles. Venereal disease, apertures, pregnancy, berdaches, morals, marriage customs, subincision, medical ethics, sexism, racism, feminism, communism, and priapism. Sikkim, Sweden, Polynesia, Melanesia, Micronesia, Indonesia, and all the tribes of Africa and Araby. Buttocks, balls, breasts, blood supplies, nervous supplies, hypothalamic supplies, gross national product, pheromones, implants, plateaus, biting, squeezing, rubbing, swinging. Nude and clothed, here and there, outlets and inlets, large and small, up and down, in and out. But not sexual excitement. Strange. (Stoller 1979, 1)

A decade and a half later, sociologist William Simon (1996, 23) wrote, "Beyond the work of Stoller and relatively few others, the question of what creates sexual excitement, how it is rooted not in our bodies but in our lives, has only been considered in the most superficial ways." Now, after yet more time—during a period in which we have seen a veritable explosion of work on so-called sexualities, as well as the creation of a new interdisciplinary field called queer theory—I'm not convinced that we know a lot more about comparative erotics. Strange.

The explanation of this lack is no doubt complex. Shame continues to play some part. But I have suggested that another reason is conceptual: however free-floating the idea of sexuality has become, it inevitably retains a central assumption that object choice trumps all other aspects of what makes sex sexy. In this way, it obscures the range of the erotic.

> The seeming simplicity and obviousness of gender create a bright light effect that either obscures other dimensions of object choice or establishes the gender of the object as the encompassing distinction that renders all other attributes subordinate... The most one can say about the dominance of gender in eliciting sexual interest or excitement is that it is a minimal precondition for most individuals most of the time, and even then not necessarily for the same reasons. The issues of age, race, physical appearance, social status, quality and history of relationship and the specifics of context, among other attributes, also play roles as compelling, if not more so, than that played by gender. (Simon 1996, 34–35)

I have suggested that we attempt to build another approach to the erotic in which the sex and gender of an object choice is seen as only another fetish—among many, many others. If there are master fetishes, this fact will only be established by an approach that does not begin with the answer it expects—and by so doing participates, itself, in the creation of "sexuality."

What made extraverted sex erotic to Africans was hardly its object (some were looking explicitly for *either* male or female foreign partners) but that it allowed an expansion of personhood via participation in a cosmopolitan world from which colonialism had previously excluded them. It also, ironically, allowed for the continuance of local kin groups. It was almost as if the erotic aroused not just the individual body but also the social body. And, of course, the "acceptance" by the ghetto itself was crucial in lessening pressures against a practice that otherwise might have drawn condemnation.

On the other side of the interaction, the white men who found their way to Africa were hardly simply "homosexuals," though they fit that category more easily than their African counterparts, and most saw themselves in such terms. They were attracted not just by *any* man, nor indeed by any *black* man. There was an element of surrender to the foreign involved, an elevation of the erotic by a degree of danger, and perhaps an aspect of enjoyable masochism—all protected by the power of a foreign passport.

Stoller provides a significantly revised version of the sexual fetish in relation to Freud:

> Let us take fetishization as the key process in the creation of erotic excitement. We might best begin by calling it dehumanization; the fetish stands for a human (not just, as is sometimes said, for a missing penis). A sexually exciting fetish, we know, may be an inanimate object, a living but not human object, a part of a human body (in rare cases even of one's own), an attribute of a human (this is a bit less sure, since we cannot hold an attribute in hand), or even a whole human not perceived as himself or herself but rather as an abstraction, such as a representative of a group rather than a person in his or her own right ("all women are bitches"; "all men are pigs"). The word "dehumanization" does not signify that the human attributes are completely removed, but just that they are reduced, letting the fetish still remind its owner of the original human connection, now repressed. As a result the same move (like a seesaw) that dehumanizes the human endows the fetish with a human quality. (Stoller 1979, 7)

The more agency attributed to a fetish, the less to the original human agent who wounded. Part of Stoller's insight involves an appreciation of the essential element of hostility. "(1) A person who has harmed one is to be punished with a similar trauma. (2) The object is stripped of its humanity. (3) A nonhuman object... is endowed with the humanness stolen from the person on whom one is to be revenged. In this way the human is dehumanized and the nonhuman humanized. (4) The fetish is chosen because it has some quality that resembles the loved, needed, traumatizing object" (Stoller 1979, 8).

But hostility can be intertwined with love: "With it [the mechanism of fetishization] one focuses on and overvalues a part without fully taking in the whole. That in itself need not, however, rule out affection. Rather than keeping two people at a distance from each other, it could be a device that, by increasing the other's erotic attractiveness, promotes closeness, enriches love" (Stoller 1979, 33).

Stoller's book, an extended account of the analysis of a woman he calls Belle, is devoted to intrapsychic conflicts. Nonetheless, as I have argued, it should provoke us to consider the other social and cultural levels at which sexual scripts are written.

Once we have constructed this approach to erotics, it is altogether striking to observe the current lopsidedness of knowledge. We know virtually nothing about the erotics of those who ostensibly do not deviate from the cultural norm, that is, the unmarked category, in the West, of straight people (see Katz 1995). That blank space arguably allows the continuing mythologization of heterosexuality.

Just as studies of race began with black people and turned to whites, and just as studies of gender started with females and moved to males, studies of the erotic need to move beyond the margins to include hegemonic forms of eroticism. I predict we are in for some surprises.

Let me consider how the approach to erotics I have been advocating differs from a focus on sexualities. Let me take up, in turn, space, time, and media.

Space. A sexuality is a state of being, and as such, it easily maps onto a picture of the world as a mosaic of differently colored, mostly internally homogeneous cultures separated by clear boundaries. Ancient Greek sexuality. Modern North American sexuality. Brazilian sexuality.

Like Ruth Benedict in *The Chrysanthemum and the Sword*, the analyst of sexualities typically oscillates back and forth between "us" and "them" (Geertz 1988) to make a thousand comparisons that finally illuminate both "them" and "us." Think of David Halperin's (1990) distinguished work on ancient Greece, *One Hundred Years of Homosexuality.*

The erotic sets up no such pressures to assume homogeneous cultural spaces (see Sedgwick 1990). The contact zone I have depicted was for centuries a blurred transitional zone between different colors on the map, an exception in a world in which the default situation was thought to be cultural homogeneity. After the Internet, the contact zone has spread out from a smudged boundary to represent something much closer to the default situation in our postmodern world.

Do not stable forms of interaction with respect to something as central as sex require shared meanings? This essay illustrates why the answer is no. Alfred Chester (1990), an American gay man writing about Paul Bowles's Tangiers, used the metaphor of a glory hole to capture the contact zone in Morocco. A glory hole, in gay terminology, is an aperture bored through a partition between stalls in a public restroom that allows for anonymous sexual intercourse. The communicating hole connects, but the partition continues to separate.

If continued interaction across cultural boundaries can eventually replace glory holes with more multidimensional interaction, in the short term the effect can be otherwise. In the ghetto described here, I would argue that the contact zone set in motion processes that depended precisely upon the maintenance—not the blurring—of cultural and linguistic boundaries. Except for Johnny, no gay white man in the ghetto, to my knowledge, learned much of the local African language.

To illustrate what I mean, consider the question of why African men were not feminized, in their own minds, by a situation in which gay Europeans were economically providing for their wives and children. Husbands do not support wives in West Africa in the same way they did at a certain point in Western history, but in patrilineal societies husbands are expected to help support children. According to this African cultural logic, why did European support for African children not threaten the masculinity of African men?

Such assuredly did not happen. It was, rather, the Europeans who were feminized by Africans, and, just like African women, they were subjected to a double standard when it came to sexual propriety. An African man might have multiple sexual partners and might have secret partners on the side (and indeed either of these could be celebrated in the right context), but if a European man attempted to do the same in Africa, he put himself in real danger and was, at the very least, morally condemned. He was a "butterfly," someone who randomly sipped from flower to flower.

So how did African men remain so male in their own terms? I would suggest that a large part of the answer rests on the fact that the two partners came from different cultural backgrounds. In a sense, this is simply a requirement of extraversion itself: an actor may "trick" outside his reference group but not inside it. If both partners were African, then the one who was supported might well have felt the pressures of feminization. For the one who was doing the supporting would have known the requisite codes, the devastating small asides, for feminizing another. This might explain the relative lack in the ghetto of eroticization of other African men, even wealthy African men.

Outside the neighborhood on which I am reporting, there were, apparently, secret underground networks of African men who had sex with other African men. According to one of the older men I interviewed in the ghetto, these relationships were focused on shrine priests of traditional religion. Same-sex sex, he contended, was the "secret" that generated the power of traditional religion.

It is interesting to note that the role of same-sex sex in African-derived religions in the New World has long been realized (Landes 1940) but that until recently, its presence on the African side has been almost totally ignored. Recently, Matory (2003) has called attention to the way that traditional spirit possession is culturally constructed in Yoruba religion. The spirit "mounts" his devotee just as a rider mounts a horse or a man sexually mounts a woman.

> Imagine my surprise when I made the acquaintance of a highly respected Yoruba art historian from Oyo, whose extended family included many Sango priests in that West African cultural capital. During his time among oricha-worshippers in the United States, this scholar too became aware of the importance of men who love men in the New World priesthoods. Without having read my work, he had concluded that male-male sexual conduct among New World priests was a continuation rather than a mere reinterpretation of West African religious traditions. He told me that, on two occasions between 1968 and 1973, he witnessed possessed male

Sango priests anally penetrate unpossessed male priests in an Oyo shrine. He does not know, however, if this practice was widespread or whether it represented a tradition or norm. Nor do I. (Matory 2003, 424)

Gay slang has long labeled the scene that Matory describes as "running a train": a deity mounts a possessed devotee, who, at the same time, mounts an unpossessed devotee. If sexual "fluidity" was a particular aspect of the ghetto, it was perhaps not absent from the wider Atlantic African cultural scene. But unlike the relationships between African and foreign men, African-African relationships were apparently closely kept secrets.

Differences in sexual cultures do not, then, necessarily mean social instability. Consider the love triangles of each of the cases I have mentioned—von Gloeden in Sicily, Bowles in Tangiers, Johnny in Atlantic Africa. The European men who successfully negotiated the contact zone in these cases did so through their "management" of love triangles. They related, in a way, to both their male lovers and their lovers' wives (and children). Triangles stabilized social interaction.

Von Gloeden kept individual accounts for each photographic image of a nude Sicilian boy he sold, and he provided royalties to the young man himself—which helped the latter marry a local woman. Bowles translated the stories of his lovers—stories about love triangles, in fact—so that they earned their own royalties. And finally, Johnny established with Justice (by then married to a second wife) a business in the ghetto that for a time created considerable support for Justice's family and, more widely, local employment.

In literary theory, there has been a long meditation on erotic triangles, the subject, after all, of countless European novels and short stories. This consideration begins (if not with Freud's

Oedipal scene of a child and a mother and father) with René Girard's description, in *Deceit, Desire, and the Novel*, of what he called mimetic desire—desire for a beloved provoked not only by the beloved but by a reaction to a rival's desire: two men attracted to the same woman. In *Between Men*, Eve Sedgwick took the argument further to examine the nature of the relationship between the two men, the creation of "homosociality," sometimes as a defense against "homosexuality." Finally, Terry Castle followed in *The Apparitional Lesbian* to analyze two women and one man, and Marjorie Garber attempted to ring all the triangular changes of gender and sexual attraction in *Bisexuality and the Eroticism of Everyday Life*. Much of the insight of this extended conversation stems from its attempts to place erotic incitement in the context of social relationality, across sexual types, not just within them.

Time. Because sexuality, unlike erotics, is figured primarily in relation to consciously held identity and therefore to political struggles, historical accounts of change in sexuality have a strong tendency to become either narratives of progress, of the past leading up to the present, or of narratives of increasing subjection (these two being mirror images of one another).

George Chauncey's work on gay marriage is a distinguished and perhaps necessary example of the first. Michel Foucault's (to retranslate the title) *The Will to Know: The History of Sexuality, Vol. 1,* is an impressive example of the second.

To follow Foucault's thought further for a moment, notice that the way he uses the notion of sexuality has little to do with sexual excitement. Indeed, in what is probably the most questionable move that Foucault makes in *The History of Sexuality, Vol. 1,* he claims that the West—unlike ancient India and Japan, for example—did not have an *ars erotica,* an art of cultivating the erotic.

"Sexuality," then, is fundamentally a matter of discourse in the context of social and political institutions, what Foucault called a *dispositif*, a device or apparatus (Halperin 1995). According to Foucault, the sexologists who thought of themselves as "discovering" homosexuality had actually created it in some senses. Ian Hacking (1984, 122) called this type of argument dynamic nominalism: "Categories of people come into existence at the same time as kinds of people come into being to fit those categories, and there is a two-way interaction between these processes." As this process works itself out, discourses in the context of social devices insert the hold of biopower ever more insidiously into acting individuals.

A turn toward erotics helps free analysis from these lines of increase or decrease. Without too much distortion, one could say that—in the imagination at least—*not all that much* changed over the centuries in the Atlantic African case I have depicted. What the Internet (re)created was simply the contact zone of previous centuries in which men from substantially different cultural points of view interacted. It is now the very idea of "sexuality"—that Europeans and Africans are alike "gay"— that functions as a fetish, just like the African ritual objects on which European and African traders took oaths centuries ago. In other words, sexuality represents now the "creative misunderstanding" that allows European-African social interaction. A certain "trade" continues, one concerned still with "gold" and sometimes even "slaves."[2]

Media. Sexuality, since it is assumed to be a state of being, a state that emanates from inside a person and that is, in fact, "discovered," does not invite questions about the role of media. In a wide-ranging study, Robert Paul (2015) has recently attempted to theorize cultural transmission per se. According to Paul, it always takes place with respect to sensory reality outside individual human beings, with language being perhaps the "first" such channel:

> ....the effective life of symbols occurs in their transmission into and through the medium of the sensory world, in the realm of things seen, heard, smelled, tasted, felt, and experienced. By virtue of being transmitted this way, rather than via copulation, symbols, unlike genes, can be perceived by and can inform many people at once, and thereby produce a sense of kinship among groups that is real in the same sense that genetic kinship is real: that is, it describes the relationship of people whose behavior is informed by the same instructions. (Paul 2015, 285)

It is far easier to pose the question of how sexual fetishes are communicated once one turns from the rubric of sexuality. Waugh points out that both homosexuality and photography were created at about the same time and have been intertwined ever since. Waugh (1996, 32) suggests that the circulation of photographs played something of the same role in shaping communities of same-sex erotics as print capitalism did with regard to nationalisms (Benedict Anderson's well-known argument). These processes are not yet fully understood. "The picture does not create desire," Simon (1996, 142) cautions, "desire creates the picture. The picture evokes desire, but only the desire that was lying in wait." One wonders whether further analysis will not grant more "agency" to images.

In any case, because of what Bazin called the "ontology" of photographs, their presumed unmediated ability not just to capture reality but to *be* real, it is clear that photographic images have an elective affinity with fetishes. And as Metz (1985) argued, because the viewer of a photograph (as opposed to a film, for example) can choose the length of time he or she gazes, photographs have the unique ability to imprint themselves on viewers. Finally, photographs viewed on a computer screen connected to the Internet add yet another layer of specificity, of assumed secrecy across wide dissemination with a shielding from public shame.

Now reproduced at virtually no cost via the span and reach of the Internet, which extends now to areas of the world like the ghetto, photographs and films have created a massive new encyclopedia of erotic reference (Escoffier 2007)—much of it beyond states' attempts to control so-called pornography. This new form of mediation allows for an explicit mobilization of erotic fetishes to an unprecedented degree and so helps to produce ever more specialized and splintered erotic communities.

As a final matter, I want to *speculate* on how fetishes—economic and erotic—interrelate in late capitalism. Let me note, first, that money may be the single object under capitalism that functions both as an economic fetish (the way it is seen misrepresents and thus preserves economic domination) and, curiously, as an erotic fetish (its contemplation can sexually arouse). Besides the materials presented here, Gregory Mitchell's (2016, 77) work on Brazilian male prostitutes who have sex with men furnishes an example: "To keep himself focused, he has the mantra that he tells himself: I want to have this money. He focuses on the money, fantasizing about cash to keep himself stimulated during the programa."

As Gayle Rubin points out in the epigraph to this book, many erotic fetishes such as latex, vinyl, and silk stockings depend upon historically particular industrial processes. They reflect a specific, capitalist history. At a deeper level, any form of power contains a kind of wounding—a dehumanization, if you will—continually recollected in both individual and collective memory. That connection is perhaps more widely appreciated in psychoanalytic approaches to the individual, but it is present as well at larger scales in both colonialism and capitalism. If Stoller, Gagnon, and Simon are correct, both colonialism and capitalism have produced their characteristic forms of erotic fetishes.

At first glance, one might assume that SM plays with and eroticizes the forms of domination found in wider society. But SM's interrelationship with capitalism is more complex than this. Indeed, it is striking, from what I can tell, that the domination of capitalists over workers is typically *not* eroticized. Why? In contrast to so-called precapitalist modes of production that name and naturalize their forms of inequality (whether that enjoyed by fathers or chiefs or feudal lords), the culture of capitalism insists that it has no domination. Workers and capitalists are formal equals. Each enters into a "free" contract. Workers sell their labor power. And capitalists buy it. In volume 1 of *Capital*, it took Marx literally hundreds of pages to demonstrate the illusion of such freedom and equality—an illusion created, Marx argued, by the fetishization of capital, the idea that money (not the labor of workers) makes money. Money can also sexually arouse, but capitalist domination itself (which is, to the degree possible, erased) cannot.

Capitalism presents itself, then, as a narrative of freedom, of a progressive removal of all previous forms of "bound" labor. But since Eric Williams's *Capitalism and Slavery* (1944), if not since Marx's own *Capital*, volume 1, we have known that things are hardly so simple. In some real sense, the Atlantic slave trade was *created* by global capitalism. After an extended and epic struggle in the nineteenth century, slavery was finally repudiated and capitalism purified to depend primarily on "free" wage labor. But then, the newly magnified shame of slavery helped to construct the increasingly unquestionable freedom of capitalism. The more shameful slavery became, the more ethically secured and egalitarian capitalism appeared. The relation between shame and labor was thus exactly reversed compared to precapitalist modes of production. In the latter, selling labor was what was shameful—that is, waged labor itself. Labor could be ethically transacted only by gifting it or by embedding it in relationships to kin or chiefs or lords (Donham [1985] 1994).

According to Tomkins, it is precisely shame that is the key affect in intrapsychic scripts of SM,[3] the practitioners of which he calls the "daredevils of shame":

> If an individual is haunted with a chronic sense of shame for sexual exploration, then the idea of power becomes necessarily tied to the violation of the constraints that originated the taboo. We have found abundant clinical evidence that under such conditions sexual excitement requires an exaggerated shamelessness or power to undo, reverse, and deny the power of the other to evoke shame for one's own sexuality. Such a one therefore becomes excited primarily by fantasies in which he, or the other, or both indulge in the most flagrant indecencies or humiliations and in which there is a reveling in shame. Other variants we have analyzed . . . include elaborate fantasies of omnipotence in which the sexual partner is a slave or a captive. (Tomkins 1995, 73–74)

So SM plays with not the actual system of domination in capitalism but its dark shadow, which, since the nineteenth century, has accompanied and defined it by contrast.[4]

In this project, it was often the details that spoke the loudest to me. Johnny once laughingly told me that when he moved from Oakland to Atlantic Africa, he had packed chains. According to African American artist Kara Walker, "Everyone wants to play the nigger now." Strategic overstatement, no doubt. But applied to the fantasies of some gay white men in Atlantic Africa, Walker's art brilliantly captures the layered, moving, and sometimes surprising nature of the erotic—a topic we scholars have hardly begun to explore.

NOTES

PREFACE

1. For Balibar on Marx, see Balibar (2017); for Foucault on the model perversion, see Foucault ([1976] 1978, 154); and for the notion of the factish, see Latour (2010).

HEADING SOUTH: AN INTRODUCTION

1. *Heading South* is the title of a 2005 film about North American female tourists to Haiti. According to the back cover of the DVD, "Disillusioned with—and unsatisfied by—the men at home, Wellesley professor Ellen (Charlotte Rampling), willowy divorcée Brenda (Karen Young) and spirited Canadian Sue (Louise Portal) soon find themselves competing for the virile Legba (Ménothy César)." Legba is the name of an African vodun deity of "trickery, communication with the gods, and sexual potency" (Blier 1995, 147).

2. Sexual systems focused on penetration were hardly unique to the Mediterranean, as shown by George Chauncey's (1985) fascinating study of a scandal at a U.S. Navy base in Rhode Island in 1919. The popular construction of male-male sex in the United States at that time—that it occurred between "queers" who allowed themselves

to be penetrated and "straights" who, for various contextual reasons, accommodated queers—was so engrained in the navy that it recruited its own seamen as undercover agents to *have* sex with queers in order to identify and eliminate the latter from the navy. Queers were seen as the only deviants in this scene. And the conceptual opposition was gender based: between effeminate males and ordinary, masculine men.

3. Class privilege typically feminized upper-class European men in relation to lower-class ones, including those in Mediterranean lands.

4. As early as the 1860s, Ulrichs wrote, "I am an insurgent. I rebel against the existing situation, because I hold it to be a condition of injustice. I fight for freedom from persecution and insults. I call for the recognition of Urning love" (quoted in H. Kennedy 1988, 70).

The designation *homosexuality* had not yet been invented, so it would be an anachronism to describe Ulrichs as homosexual. Rather, Ulrichs saw himself and others as souls of women trapped in men's bodies. Like women, Urnings' "natural" attraction was to men, ordinary men—not other Urnings—the iconic attraction being young soldiers. Thus, such attraction could never be "unnatural," and because it was inborn, according to Ulrich, and not subject to choice and thereby responsibility, it should not be legally punished.

Notice the role of "choice" or its lack here. As others have emphasized, the relationship between the view that homosexuality is biologically given and therefore not subject to choice can either make it easier for people to accept (as in the late twentieth-century United States) or justify the opposite reaction of elimination (as in Nazi Germany). Janet E. Halley's (1993–94) work is a brilliant critique of legal strategies that rely solely on the notion of lack of choice.

5. See Eve Sedgwick and Adam Frank's (1995) meditation on shame in the work of Silvan Tomkins.

6. For an excellent analysis of Africa's assumed "heterosexuality," see Epprecht (2008). Recent collections on queer Africa include Tamale (2011), Ekine and Abbas (2013), and Nyeck and Epprecht (2013). On Islamic lands, see El-Rouayheb (2005).

7. See Kate Murphy, "Seeking Love, Getting Scammed," *New York Times,* January 17, 2016, Sunday Review section, 4.

8. Something of the same kind of reversal, with respect to gender rather than race, occurs when a dominatrix carries out her magic.

9. "All too often, psychoanalysis has been relegated to the (conventionally universal) realm of private, domestic space, while politics and economics are relegated to the (conventionally historical) realm of the public market. I argue that the disciplinary quarantine of psychoanalysis from history was germane to imperial modernity itself" (McClintock 1995, 8). The Munby-Cullwick relationship has provoked a flood of articles and books (see Reay 2002 for a bibliography).

10. The sexual fluidity of women, in the United States at least, is apparently easier to admit and therefore to analyze than that of men (see Diamond 2008). Part of the attraction of the concept of sexuality in the United States may be, then, precisely that it shores up a certain construction of male gender. In the analysis to follow, African men married to African women, in contrast, had no problem in having exuberant sex, apparently of all kinds, with European men.

11. See Gayle Rubin's essay, "Geologies of Queer Studies: It's Déjà Vu All Over Again," in her collected essays. "The more I explore these queer knowledges, the more I find out how much we have already forgotten, rediscovered, and promptly forgotten again. I myself have attempted to reinvent the wheel on several occasions" (Rubin 2011, 327).

12. In relation to Foucault's account of the sexual scientists of the late nineteenth century, it is interesting to note that Kinsey's "will to know" apparently accomplished the opposite of what Foucault claimed to have occurred in the nineteenth century: it "deconstructed" sexuality.

Kinsey found, famously, of North American males in the 1940s that at least 37 percent had had some homosexual experience to the point of orgasm over the course of their lives. Kinsey was maniacally devoted to the statistical tabulation of behavior. Here, I am concerned to take behavior into account, but I want to attend to the meanings that actors and observers attribute to behaviors, as these meanings are transmitted via various media.

13. See Wiegman (2015) on the way that antinormativity has, so far, constituted queer theory. The question of just what the norm is becomes determinative, then, for any antinormative analysis. Paul

(2015) argues that biological reproduction, by itself, has never been the norm in human societies.

14. My argument at this point parallels some of the claims of David Graeber (2005, 430) about the fetish in relation to economic exchange: "Even when fetishes were not explicitly about establishing contracts of one sort or another, they were almost invariably the basis for creating something new: congregations, new social relations, new communities. Hence any 'totality' involved was, at least at first, virtual, imaginary, and prospective. What is more—and this is the really crucial point—it was an imaginary totality that could only come into real existence if everyone acted as if the fetish object actually did have subjective qualities."

15. The difference that homosexual rights made in the lives of North American men and women in the twentieth century is vividly captured by Esther Newton's social history, *Cherry Grove, Fire Island* (1993).

16. Latour is not concerned with sexual fetishes per se and often seems more concerned with the Marxist than the Freudian version.

17. By *gay* or *queer*, I mean only that set of persons who identify as such.

18. Gregory Mitchell's *Tourist Attractions* is a notable exception to this tendency. At one point, Mitchell writes, "there is danger to feminist and queer approaches that cast professional intellectuals in the role of restricting the sexuality of other people, foreclosing (sometimes with eager and righteous indignation) the sexual choices and erotic possibilities of others" (2016, 67).

19. Some time ago (Donham 1990, 196–205), I argued that a simplified construction of love functions precisely to naturalize wage labor. Love is defined, as David Schneider (1980) argued for North American kinship, as "what money can't buy." While that definition captures the symbolic oppositions of Western ideology, nowhere does it describe love's social reality. One only has to appreciate the rate of class endogamy, heterosexual or homosexual, to appreciate that fact. Real love has its economic underpinnings and requirements.

Why can't we pose the question of the morality of selling labor power? Is it because, among other reasons, we already assume the immorality of selling sex?

CHAPTER ONE

1. Johnny did not like being described as a fetishist, since to him it seemed necessarily to connote a one-sided and exploitative sexual relationship that he had taken care to avoid. The latter, as will become clear below, is not my idea of fetishism. For me, the fetish underlies all sexual desire.

2. The notion of "homophobia" in Africa has grown almost stereotypic in Western media. See the excellent ethnographic analysis of Awondo, Geschiere, and Reid (2012) and the legal and human rights perspective of Ugandan lawyer Sylvia Tamale (2013). For the very different case of Thailand, see Morris's insightful essay (1997).

3. In 2005 Newell interviewed the nephew of Stuart-Young's first African lover. According to the nephew, "Stuart-Young just landed and then perched in Onitsha. He did not like women much. My uncle consulted him if he had a problem, and he consulted my uncle. He helped my uncle, in fact he was a part of the family." Stuart-Young didn't give his uncle "any trouble, but people began to be anxious. He doesn't mix up much. We have so many gossips. I can't say what they were accusing him of" (2006, 81).

4. Later I realized that there were at least two publications on Atlantic African social scenes close to the one I had discovered. The first is Nii Ajen (129–38) in Stephen O. Murray and Will Roscoe's pioneering 1998 volume, *Boy-Wives and Female Husbands: Studies in African Homosexualities*. Ajen concludes, "On the whole, what this essay underscores is the need for more of us to undertake research on same-sex love in non-Western cultures" (138). The other is Vinh-Kim Nguyen's 2005 chapter in Vincanne Adams and Stacey Pigg's edited collection *Sex in Development: Science, Sexuality and Morality in a Global Perspective*.

5. One of Nguyen's (2005, 252) African informants in Abidjan called men who had sex with both men and women "economic bisexuals." But Nguyen (2005, 253) concluded, "Homosexual relations could not be reduced to economic strategy nor were they simply about experimenting with gender roles. Rather, as forms of self-fashioning they incorporated concerns that were simultaneously those of material and emotional satisfaction, pleasure and desire."

6. I was questioned repeatedly in 2012 about just which states in the United States had gay marriage—a measure of just how involved young Africans were in the details of North American life. They were quite aware of the legal desirability of marriage.

7. Various kinds of scams have become endemic to West Africa during the last two decades. See, for example, Daniel J. Smith's (2007) work on everyday life in Nigeria and Charles Piot's (2010) description of how Western visas are obtained in Ghana and Togo.

8. The connections between various kinds of travel and same-sex sex are deep (Hilderbrand 2013), sometimes, as with "slumming," involving only movement across racial and class boundaries of the same city (Heap 2009; Herring 2007; Koven 2004).

9. Sex was a part of the informal economy described by Hart, for both women and men. "Some young men receive payment in cash or kind as the sexual partners to older, prosperous women" (1973, 76).

CHAPTER TWO

1. "We find copies of the French edition [of Bosman's book] in the libraries of Newton and Locke and a copy of the English version in Gibbon's library. It is not listed among Adam Smith's books, but Smith had a thorough knowledge of the text and refers to it a number of times" (Pietz 1988, 117).

2. Paul Morrison (1993, 55) writes of Freud, "Like the well-made narrative, normative sexual activity issues in climax from which comes, as it were, quiescence; like the well-made narrative, moreover, normative sexuality is end-haunted, all for its end. The perversions of adults . . . are intelligible only as 'the sickness of uncompleted narratives'." See, however, the more complex exposition of Freud—one that reads Freud's contradictions—by Arnold Davidson (1987, 263–67). I have assumed here that a version of Freud without reproductive teleology, a postmodern Freud, is possible, though I have not presented it here.

3. By "disavowal," Freud meant the state in which an individual simultaneously holds contradictory beliefs.

4. Henry Krips (1999, 89) has argued that Lacan's work adds to Freud's story of the fetish additional insights into desire and plea-

sure. "A three-cornered game involving a *subject*, and object of desire, and a little 'other object,' what Lacan calls *objet petit autre* (*objet a* for short), which stands in the way of subjects getting what they want. Engaging this little other object, circling it, affords subjects a degree of pleasure—it 'goes some way to satisfying the pleasure principle'— and thus distracts them from their continuing state of lack." According to Krips, fetishes are a kind of *objet a*.

5. This story obviously implies that women cannot have fetishes— something we know is false. Feminism since Freud has been both inspired and exasperated by him. See Elizabeth Grosz (1993). Sander Gilman presents a fascinating interpretation of the effects of racial stereotypes of Jews, particularly of Eastern Jews, on Freud's (displaced) view of women. "The image of the clitoris as a 'truncated penis,' as a less than intact penis, reflects the popular *fin-de-siècle* Viennese view of the relationship between the body of the male Jew and the body of the woman. The clitoris was known in Viennese slang of the *fin de siècle* simply as 'Jew' *(Jud)*" (Gilman 1994, 342).

6. Jean-Martin Charcot and Valentin Magnan (1882).

7. The role of the sexual scientists in "creating" sexual identities can be overstated (see Oosterhuis 1997). The sexologists, in fact, picked up concepts like "inversion" from the sexual underground (see the case of Karl Heinrich Ulrichs, described by H. Kennedy 1988 and Beachy 2014). Later, when sexologists invented new categories like homo- and heterosexuality, it sometimes took many decades for the lower classes to be affected. For some of the historical complexities, see Chauncey (1983) and Duggan (2000).

8. Edelman's *No Future* is a polemic against what I am calling teleology and what he calls "reproductive futurism." He attempts to construct an effective politics to combat it: "Rather than rejecting, with liberal discourse, this ascription of negativity to the queer, we might, as I argue, do better to consider accepting and even embracing it" (2004, 4). As will be clear by the end of this work, I am not convinced that the alternatives that Edelman sees are the only ones.

9. Lest I participate in a naive narrative of "progress," I would point out that repression of some of the nineteenth-century perversions, such as intergenerational sex, hardened and sometimes grew

outright hysterical. Was there some necessary relationship between the redistribution of the perversions?

CHAPTER FOUR

1. What straight men do and do not do is, of course, strictly historically and situationally bound. A striking example is provided by Reay (2010), who shows that masculine male hustlers in New York City were typically straight well into the twentieth century, up to the beginnings of gay liberation in the 1970s. By "straight," I mean identity and preference as these are experienced by social actors.

2. As a measure of just how misleading the notion of sexuality can become and with what real consequences, ponder Catharine MacKinnon's (1989, 3) famous declaration: "Sexuality is to feminism what work is to Marxism: that which is most one's own, yet most taken away."

3. This point *was* argued by Mary McIntosh (1968). According to Jeffrey Weeks (1998, 139), "Foucault's *The History of Sexuality* is often seen, misleadingly, as the locus classicus of approaches that attribute the emergence of the homosexual category in the nineteenth century to medicalization. But the agenda on this was already set by McIntosh, as was the question of the impact of would-be medical definitions on individual lives."

4. According to Kunzel (2008, 237), "Prison is but one locus from which modern sexuality has been confounded and destabilized by sexual acts, desires, and identities that failed (and fail) to map clearly onto categories of 'gay' or 'straight.' Their long history suggests that the homo/heterosexual binary was not only 'stunningly recent,' as George Chauncey so provocatively and generatively proposed, but that it was also remarkably uneven and considerably less hegemonic and less coherent than historians have often assumed."

5. Theoretical arguments that attempt to depart in some fundamental way from conventional wisdom always face the issue of whether to ban old terms or to try to repurpose them. My inclination at every juncture has been to try to replace the word "sexuality" by a more precise description of what I am trying to argue. That always clarifies, I believe.

But another strategy would be to attempt to redefine "sexuality" as the virtually unique and changing array of sexual fetishes that a person accumulates over a particular lifetime in a specific cultural location during a specific historical period. Such could include "the vibration of your car," as well as "your unconscious wish to sleep with your mother and kill your father" (Halley 2006, 24). Both of these fetishes set up some degree of temporal durability. "You could want to be turned on by the vibration of your car *one more time*" (24). If so, this description would repurpose "sexuality" in the terms I'm trying to develop in this essay. But I believe "sexuality" has been too deeply sedimented into our collective conscience for that strategy to be successful.

CHAPTER FIVE

1. This paragraph is based on numerous authors, the most famous of whom is, of course, Frantz Fanon ([1952] 2008). See also Calvin Hernton (1965) and, among others, Sander Gilman (1985b) and Richard Fung (1991). Robert A. Paul (n.d.) formed my analysis of these issues.

Katsuhiko Suganuma's (2012) excellent study, *Contact Moments*, is, in many ways, the mirror image of the case I describe here, the queer contact zone between (feminized) Japanese and whites.

See also John Whittier Treat (1999, x) who argues that *all* study of other cultures participates in the processes of the contact zone: "The student of another culture who travels there goes thinking: I will watch how those people live, or work, or write, and then bring their lessons home. But he goes abroad as a man or woman, and so with his intellectual intents goes too a sexual body. His desire for knowledge is easily confused with his desire to possess or be possessed by other things: passion. The body becomes his methodology, and his desire for union an epistemology."

2. Early twentieth-century sexologist Iwan Bloch (1933, 72) wrote, "The savage carves obscene images of wood which are to inflame the libido at erotic festivals; civilized man has invented obscene photography, which serves the same ultimate purpose." I'm not certain that Bloch understood the "savage" world, but clearly he was calling attention to the role of photography in his own world.

The attractions of photography to fetishists like Arthur J. Munby, Carl Van Vechten, Leni Riefenstahl, and Robert Mapplethorpe are evident. Not only that, but the preservation of a photographic archive, sure to be misunderstood in its own time, in a place of elevated cultural value (Munby's at Trinity College and Van Vechten's at Yale University) seems noteworthy. By Mapplethorpe's day, the evidence of the fetish did not need to be discreetly archived. It could be commercially exploited.

3. The Robert Mapplethorpe Foundation turned down my request to reproduce *Man in Polyester Suit*.

4. Barthes ([1980] 1981, 59) offered this rather high-minded discussion of pornography: "Pornography ordinarily represents the sexual organs, making them into a motionless object (a fetish), flattered like an idol that does not leave its niche; for me, there is no punctum in the pornographic image; at most it amuses me (and even then, boredom follows quickly)."

CHAPTER SEVEN

1. The Internet is changing not just sex; it is changing ethnography as well. For another demonstration of this, see James Smith and Ngeti Mwadime's *Email from Ngeti* (2014).

2. In what follows, I rely principally on Gayle Rubin, "Valley of the Kings: Leathermen in San Francisco, 1960–1990" (PhD diss., University of Michigan, Department of Anthropology, 1994).

3. Through their very theatricality, hypermasculine styles always hold the potential to deconstruct: "The butch number swaggering into a bar in a leather get-up opens his mouth and sounds like a pansy, takes you home, where the first thing you notice is the complete work of Jane Austen, gets you into bed, and—well, you know the rest....In short, the mockery of gay machismo is almost exclusively an internal affair, and it is based on the dark suspicion that you may not be getting the real article" (Bersani 1987, 208).

This reaction captured the view of Samuel Steward, for example, who had been involved in violent erotic encounters with straight men since the 1930s: "As leather had evolved into a social movement during the late 1950s, Steward had assiduously avoided its gatherings, remaining skeptical not only of its emerging rites and rituals but also of the masculinity of its adherents. To the end of his life, Steward would maintain that it was impossible to institutionalize a sexual practice that was, to his mind, based on the propositioning of rough, dangerous, potentially violent working-class or criminal-class men. This pursuit and seduction of an authentically masculine, primarily heterosexual, and barely civilized ideal was, to Steward's mind, essentially a solitary practice" (Spring 2010, 301).

4. It is noteworthy, as Robert Bienvenu and Gayle Rubin emphasize, that leather was a new twentieth-century fetish. It does not appear in Krafft-Ebing's late nineteenth-century compilation, for example, where, as we have seen, many others are catalogued, like aprons, feathers, undergarments, gloves, silk, and velvet. See Robert V. Bienvenu II, "The Development of Sadomasochism as a Cultural Style in the Twentieth-Century United States" (PhD diss., Indiana University, Department of Sociology, 1998).

Bienvenu built on anthropologist Paul Gebbard, who pointed out:

> Hard fetish objects are generally smooth, slick, and with a hard metallic sheen. Leather, rubber, and lately plastics, exemplify this. Hard fetish items are often tight constricting garments or shoes, usually black. Note that in our culture a tight black shiny dress is regarded as the trademark of the *femme fatale*. Hard media fetishism very frequently is associated with sadomasochism. In other cases the hard media fetishist in his or her garb feels secure and armored against the world, much like matron who feels soft and vulnerable without her corset or the military officer who feels ineffectual out of uniform. Soft media fetish objects are fluffy, frilly, or soft in texture. Fur and lingerie are common examples. There is no emphasis on constriction or tightness. Color is generally less important . . . (Gebbard 1976, 159)

5. Such a shift also took place in Robert Mapplethorpe's photographic obsessions, as he turned from the theatrics of SM to an idealization of the black male body.

6. Was this passage in fact written by a white slave for a black master's profile so that he could attract more slaves? Professional "typists" like the one Justice hired kept actual libraries of profiles for their clients.

CONCLUSION

1. Scholars have recently attempted to focus on "affect" as such (see Gregg and Seigworth 2010). As the authors note, it is often difficult to "separate out" affect from its contexts. I have sought to embed an analysis of the passions in their opposition to "rationality," or to use Albert Hirschman's terms, the passions and the interests, since these two, as I have argued, seem to constitute one another in the West.

2. There were, of course, critical material changes along the coast during this period.

3. This is the essential point that reactions against SM typically do not appreciate. It is the shame of Nazi symbols, CIA interrogations, and racialized slavery that participants seem to seek—not their politics. The erotic is related—not reducible—to political economy. When participants in SM rituals repeat, rather than invert, the raced domination of actual historical slavery, the affects produced can be exquisitely complicated. Gary Fisher was an African American graduate student living in San Francisco during the 1980s, a man intensely sexually aroused by serving "cruel" white masters. In Fisher's (1996, 236) diary, edited by Eve Sedgwick, he worries about whether his "kinky sexual gratification [was] built on and fueled by self-hatred…but which came first: the sex or the hatred?" But then he immediately goes on to add, "Indeed, I believe it was none of the above. It was FEAR. Fear of being hurt (because I was black).…"

4. Elizabeth Freeman offers a compelling interpretation of Isaac Julien's *The Attendant* that focuses on temporality. As in a long and distinguished leftist tradition of sex thought, she offers what I would call a weak redemptive reading of SM (Freeman 2008, 34, 63). Whether or not SM offers some liberatory impulse in our (capitalist) present I cannot decide. That it offers an intense form of eroticism and pleasure for some is, on the other hand, clear.

BIBLIOGRAPHY

Abelove, Henry, Michèle Aina Barale, and David M. Halperin, eds. 1993. *The Lesbian and Gay Studies Reader.* New York: Routledge.
Ades, Dawn. 1995. "Surrealism: Fetishism's Job." In *Fetishism: Visualising Power and Desire,* edited by Anthony Shelton, 67–87. London: South Bank Centre and Brighton: The Royal Pavilion, Art Gallery, and Museums.
Ahmed, Sara. 2006. *Queer Phenomenology: Orientations, Objects, Others.* Durham: Duke University Press.
Ajen, Nii. 1998. "West African Homoeroticism: West African Men Who Have Sex with Men." In *Boy-Wives and Female Husbands: Studies in African Homosexualities,* edited by Stephen O. Murray and Will Roscoe, 129–38. New York: Palgrave.
Aldrich, Robert. 2003. *Colonialism and Homosexuality.* London: Routledge.
Allen, Samantha. n.d. *Unfit to Print: A Textual History of Sexual Fetishism in the 20th Century—A Review Essay for the Kinsey Institute for Research in Sex, Gender and Reproduction.*
Apter, Emily, and William Pietz, eds. 1993. *Fetishism as Cultural Discourse.* Ithaca: Cornell University Press.
Atkinson, Diane. 2003. *Love and Dirt: The Marriage of Arthur Munby and Hannah Cullwick.* London: Pan Books.

Awondo, Patrick, Peter Geschiere, and Graeme Reid. 2012. "Homophobic Africa? Toward a More Nuanced View." *African Studies Review* 55 (3): 145–68.

Balibar, Étienne. 2017. *The Philosophy of Marx*. Updated new ed. London: Verso.

Ballantyne, Tony, and Antoinette Burton, eds. 2005. *Bodies in Contact: Rethinking Colonial Encounters in World History*. Durham: Duke University Press.

Banks, William D. 2011. "'This Thing Is Sweet': Ntetee and the Reconfiguration of Sexual Subjectivity in Post-Colonial Ghana." *Ghana Studies* 14: 265–90.

———. 2012. "Remembering Okomfo Kwabene: 'Motherhood,' Spirituality and Queer Leadership in Ghana." *African Historical Review* 44 (2): 1–17.

Barthes, Roland. (1980) 1981. *Camera Lucida*. Translated by Richard Howard. New York: Hill and Wang.

Basu, Biman. 2012. *The Commerce of People: Sadomasochism and African American Literature*. Lanham, MD: Lexington Books.

Bataille, Georges. (1957) 1986. *Erotism: Death and Sensuality*. Translated by Mary Dalwood. San Francisco: City Lights Books.

Bayart, Jean-François. (1989) 1993. *The State in Africa: The Politics of the Belly*. Cambridge: Polity Press.

———. 2000. "Africa and the World: A History of Extraversion." *African Affairs* 99: 217–67.

Baym, Nancy K. 2010. *Personal Connections in the Digital Age*. Cambridge: Polity Press.

Bazin, André. 1967. *What Is Cinema?* Translated by Hugh Gray. Berkeley: University of California Press.

Beachy, Robert. 2014. *Gay Berlin: Birthplace of a Modern Identity*. New York: Alfred A. Knopf.

Belting, Hans. (2001) 2011. *An Anthropology of Images: Picture, Medium, Body*. Translated by Thomas Dunlap. Princeton: Princeton University Press.

Berlant, Lauren. 2014. "Desire" and "Love." In *Critical Terms for the Study of Gender*, edited by Catharine R. Stimpson and Gilbert Herdt, 66–96, 250–70. Chicago: University of Chicago Press.

Bersani, Leo. 1987. "Is the Rectum a Grave?" *AIDS: Cultural Analysis/Cultural Activism* 43: 197–222.

———. 1995. "Foucault, Freud, Fantasy, and Power." *GLQ: A Journal of Lesbian and Gay Studies* 2: 11–33.

Binet, Alfred. 1887. "Le fétichisme dans l'amour: Etude de psychologie morbide." *Revue philosophique* 24: 143–67, 252–74.

Binnie, Jon. 2004. *The Globalization of Sexuality*. London: Sage.

Bleys, Rudi. 1995. *The Geography of Perversion: Male-to-Male Sexual Behavior Outside the West and the Ethnographic Imagination, 1750–1918*. New York: New York University Press.

Blier, Suzanne Preston. 1995. *African Vodun: Art, Psychology, and Power*. Chicago: University of Chicago Press.

Bloch, Iwan. 1933. *Strange Sexual Practices of All Races in All Ages*. Translated by Keene Wallis. New York: Anthropological Press.

Boone, Joseph A. 1995. "Vacation Cruises: Or, The Homoerotics of Orientalism." *PMLA* 110 (1): 89–107.

———. 1998. *Libidinal Currents: Sexuality and the Shaping of Modernism*. Chicago: University of Chicago Press.

———. 2014. *The Homoerotics of Orientalism*. New York: Columbia University Press.

Brennan, Denise. 2004. *What's Love Got to Do with It? Transnational Desires and Sex Tourism in the Dominican Republic*. Durham: Duke University Press.

Bristow, Joseph. 1998. "Symond's History, Ellis's Heredity: Sexual Inversion." In *Sexology in Culture: Labelling Bodies and Desires*, edited by Lucy Bland and Laura Doan, 79–99. Cambridge: Polity Press.

Brooks, George E. 2003. *Eurafricans in Western Africa: Commerce, Social Status, Gender, and Religious Observance from the Sixteenth to the Eighteenth Century*. Athens: Ohio University Press.

Buck-Morss, Susan. 2000. *Dreamworld and Catastrophe: The Passing of Mass Utopia in East and West*. Cambridge: MIT Press.

Burrell, Jenna. 2012. *Invisible Users: Youth in the Internet Cafés of Urban Ghana*. Cambridge: MIT Press.

Butler, Judith. 1993. "The Lesbian Phallus and the Morphological Imaginary." In *Bodies That Matter: On the Discursive Limits of "Sex,"* 57–91. New York: Routledge.

Castle, Terry. 1993. *The Apparitional Lesbian: Female Homosexuality and Modern Culture.* New York: Columbia University Press.
Charcot, Jean-Martin, and Valentin Magnan. 1882. "Inversion du sens genital." *Archives de neurologie* (3 & 4): 53–60 and 296–322.
Chauncey, George. 1983. "From Sexual Inversion to Homosexuality: Medicine and the Changing Conceptualization of Female Deviance." *Salmagundi* 58/59: 114–46.
———. 1985. "Christian Brotherhood or Sexual Perversion? Homosexual Identities and the Construction of Sexual Boundaries in the World War I Era." *Journal of Social History* 19: 189–212.
Chernoff, John M. 2003. *Hustling Is Not Stealing: Stories of an African Bar Girl.* Chicago: University of Chicago Press.
Chester, Alfred. 1990. "Glory Hole." In *Head of a Sad Angel: Stories 1953–1966,* 217–31. Santa Rosa, CA: Black Sparrow Press.
Cole, Jennifer. 2010. *Sex and Salvation: Imagining the Future in Madagascar.* Chicago: University of Chicago Press.
Cole, Jennifer, and Lynn M. Thomas, eds. 2009. *Love in Africa.* Chicago: University of Chicago Press.
Constable, Nicole. 2009. "The Commodification of Intimacy: Marriage, Sex, and Reproductive Labor." *Annual Review of Anthropology* 38: 49–64.
Crompton, Louis. 1985. *Byron and Greek Love: Homophobia in 19th-Century England.* Berkeley: University of California Press.
Cruz-Malavé, Arnaldo, and Martin F. Manalansan IV. 2002. *Queer Globalizations: Citizenship and the Afterlife of Colonialism.* New York: New York University Press.
Davidoff, Lenore. 1974. "Mastered for Life: Servant and Wife in Victorian and Edwardian England." *Journal of Social History* 7 (4): 406–28.
———. 1979. "Class and Gender in Victorian England: The Diaries of Arthur J. Munby and Hannah Cullwick." *Feminist Studies* 5 (1): 87–141.
Davidson, Arnold I. 1987. "How to Do the History of Psychoanalysis: A Reading of Freud's 'Three Essays on the Theory of Sexuality.'" *Critical Inquiry* 13 (2): 252–77.
———. 2001. *The Emergence of Sexuality: Historical Epistemology and the Formation of Concepts.* Cambridge: Harvard University Press.

Dean, Tim. 2000. *Beyond Sexuality.* Chicago: University of Chicago Press.

Diamond, Lisa M. 2008. *Sexual Fluidity: Understanding Women's Love and Desire.* Cambridge: Harvard University Press.

Donham, Donald L. (1985) 1994. *Work and Power in Maale, Ethiopia.* 2nd ed. New York: Columbia University Press.

―――. 1990. *History, Power, Ideology: Central Issues in Marxism and Anthropology.* 2nd ed. Berkeley: University of California Press.

―――. 1998. "Freeing South Africa: The 'Modernization' of Male-Male Sexuality in Soweto." *Cultural Anthropology* 13 (1): 3–21.

―――. 2011. *Violence in a Time of Liberation: Murder and Ethnicity at a South African Gold Mine, 1994.* Durham: Duke University Press.

Dorjahn, V.R., and Christopher Fyfe. 1962. "Landlord and Stranger: Change in Tenancy Relations in Sierra Leone." *Journal of African History* 3 (3): 391–97.

Duggan, Lisa. 2000. *Sapphic Slashers: Sex, Violence, and American Modernity.* Durham: Duke University Press.

Ebron, Paulla. 1997. "Traffic in Men." In *Gendered Encounters: Challenging Cultural Boundaries and Social Hierarchies in Africa,* edited by Maria Grosz-Ngate and Omari H. Kokole, 223–44. New York: Routledge.

Edelman, Lee. 2004. *No Future: Queer Theory and the Death Drive.* Durham: Duke University Press.

Ekine, Sokari, and Hakima Abbas, eds. 2013. *Queer African Reader.* Dakar: Pambazuka Press.

Elhaik, Tarek. 2008. "Anthropology and Images: Pedagogical Notes on Cinematic Boudoirs." *La critica sociologica* 42: 49–59.

―――. 2016. *The Incurable-Image: Curating Post-Mexican Film and Media Arts.* Edinburgh: Edinburgh University Press.

Ellis, Havelock. 1908. *Sexual Inversion. Studies in the Psychology of Sex,* vol. 2. 2nd ed. Philadelphia: F.A. Davis Co.

El-Rouayheb, Khaled. 2005. *Before Homosexuality in the Arab-Islamic World, 1500–1800.* Chicago: University of Chicago Press.

Eng, David L. 2001. *Racial Castration: Managing Masculinity in Asian America.* Durham: Duke University Press.

Epprecht, Marc. 2008. *Heterosexual Africa? The History of an Idea from the Age of Exploration to the Age of AIDS.* Athens: Ohio University Press.

Escoffier, Jeffrey. 2007. "Scripting the Sex: Fantasy, Narrative, and Sexual Scripts in Pornographic Films." In *The Sexual Self: The Construction of Sexual Scripts,* edited by Michael Kimmel, 61–79. Nashville: Vanderbilt University Press.

Faier, Lieba, and Lisa Rofel. 2014. "Ethnographies of Encounter." *Annual Review of Anthropology* 43: 363–77.

Fanon, Frantz. (1952) 2008. *Black Skin, White Masks.* Translated by Richard Philcox. New York: Grove Press.

Ferguson, Roderick A. 2004. *Aberrations in Black: Toward a Queer of Color Critique.* Minneapolis: University of Minnesota Press.

Fisher, Gary. 1996. *Gary in Your Pocket: Stories and Notebooks of Gary Fisher.* Edited by Eve Kosofsky Sedgwick. Durham: Duke University Press.

Foucault, Michel. (1976) 1978. *The History of Sexuality, Vol. 1: An Introduction.* Translated by Robert Hurley. New York: Vintage Books.

Freeman, Elizabeth. 2008. "Turn the Beat Around: Sadomasochism, Temporality, History." *differences* 19 (1): 32–67.

Freud, Sigmund. (1925, 6th ed.) 2000. *Three Essays on the Theory of Sexuality.* Translated by James Strachey. New York: Basic Books.

Fung, Richard. 1991. "Looking for My Penis." In *How Do I Look? Queer Film and Video,* edited by Bad Object-Choices, 145–68. Seattle: Bay Press.

Furet, François. (1995) 1999. *The Passing of an Illusion: The Idea of Communism in the Twentieth Century.* Translated by Deborah Furet. Chicago: University of Chicago Press.

Gagnon, John H., and William Simon. (1973) 2005. *Sexual Conduct: The Social Sources of Human Sexuality.* 2nd ed. New York: Aldine de Gruyter.

Garber, Marjorie. 2000. *Bisexuality and the Eroticism of Everyday Life.* New York: Routledge.

Gebbard, Paul H. 1976. "Fetishism and Sadomasochism." In *Sex Research: Studies from the Kinsey Institute,* edited by Martin S. Weinberg, 156–66. New York: Oxford University Press.

Geertz, Clifford. 1973. *The Interpretation of Cultures.* New York: Basic Books.

———. 1988. *Works and Lives: The Anthropologist as Author.* Stanford: Stanford University Press.

Gilman, Sander L. 1985a. *Difference and Pathology: Stereotypes of Sexuality, Race, and Madness.* Ithaca: Cornell University Press.

———. 1985b. "Black Bodies, White Bodies: Toward an Iconography of Female Sexuality in Late Nineteenth Century Art, Medicine, and Literature." *Critical Inquiry* 12 (l): 204–42.

———. 1994. "Sigmund Freud and the Sexologists: A Second Reading." In *Sexual Knowledge, Sexual Science: The History of Attitudes to Sexuality*, edited by Roy Porter and Mikulas Teich, 323–49. Cambridge: Cambridge University Press.

Girard, René. (1961) 1966. *Deceit, Desire, and the Novel: Self and Other in Literary Structure*. Translated by Yvonne Freccero. Baltimore: Johns Hopkins University Press.

Gordon, Robert. 1998. "The Rise of the Bushman Penis: Germans, Genitalia and Genocide." *African Studies* 57 (1): 27–34.

Gosselin, Chris, and Glenn Wilson. 1980. *Sexual Variations: Fetishism, Sadomasochism, and Transvestism*. New York: Simon and Schuster.

Graeber, David. 2005. "Fetishism as Social Creativity: or, Fetishes Are Gods in the Process of Construction." *Anthropological Theory* 5 (4): 407–38.

———. 2015. "Radical Alterity Is Just Another Way of Saying 'Reality': A Reply to Eduardo Viveiros de Castro." *Hau: Journal of Ethnographic Theory* 5 (2): 1–41.

Gregg, Melissa, and Gregory J. Seigworth, eds. 2010. *The Affect Theory Reader*. Durham: Duke University Press.

Grinker, Roy Richard. 2000. *In the Arms of Africa: The Life of Colin M. Turnbull*. Chicago: University of Chicago Press.

Grosz, Elizabeth. 1993. "Lesbian Fetishism?" In *Fetishism as Cultural Discourse*, edited by Emily Apter and William Pietz, 101–15. Ithaca: Cornell University Press.

Guyer, Jane I. 1993. "Wealth in People and Self-Realisation in Equatorial Africa." *Man* 28 (2): 243–65.

———. 2004. *Marginal Gains: Monetary Transactions in Atlantic Africa*. Chicago: University of Chicago Press.

Hacking, Ian. 1984. "Five Parables." In *Philosophy in History*, edited by Richard Rorty, J.B. Schneewind, and Quentin Skinner, 103–24. Cambridge: Cambridge University Press.

———. 1986. "Making Up People." In *Reconstructing Individualism*, edited by Thomas C. Heller, Morton Sosna, and David E. Wellbery, 161–71. Stanford: Stanford University Press.

Halley, Janet. 1993–94. "Sexual Orientation and the Politics of Biology: A Critique of the Argument from Immutability." *Stanford Law Review* 46 (3): 503–68.

———. 2006. *Split Decisions: How and Why to Take a Break from Feminism.* Princeton: Princeton University Press.

Halperin, David M. 1990. *One Hundred Years of Homosexuality and Other Essays on Greek Love.* New York: Routledge.

———. 1995. *Saint Foucault: Towards a Gay Hagiography.* New York: Oxford University Press.

———. 2002. *How to Do the History of Homosexuality.* Chicago: University of Chicago Press.

———. 2003. "The Normalization of Queer Theory." *Journal of Homosexuality* 45 (2–4): 339–43.

Hart, Keith. 1973. "Informal Income Opportunities and Urban Employment in Ghana." *Journal of Modern African Studies* 11 (1): 61–89.

Harvey, David. 1990. *The Condition of Postmodernity.* Oxford: Blackwell Publishers.

Heap, Chad. 2009. *Slumming: Sexual and Racial Encounters in American Nightlife, 1885–1940.* Chicago: University of Chicago Press.

Hendriks, Thomas. 2014. "Race and Desire in the Porno-Tropics: Ethnographic Perspectives from the Post-Colony." *Sexualities* 17 (1/2): 213–29.

Hernton, Calvin C. 1965. *Sex and Racism in America.* New York: Anchor Books.

Herring, Scott. 2007. *Queering the Underworld: Slumming, Literature, and the Undoing of Lesbian and Gay History.* Chicago: University of Chicago Press.

Hilderbrand, Lucas. 2013. "A Suitcase Full of Vaseline, or Travels in the 1970s Gay World." *Journal of the History of Sexuality* 23 (3): 373–402.

Hirschfeld, Magnus. (1920) 2000. *The Homosexuality of Men and Women.* Translated by Michael A. Lombardi-Nash. Amherst, NY: Prometheus Books.

Hirschman, Albert. 1977. *The Passions and the Interests: Political Arguments for Capitalism before Its Triumph.* Princeton: Princeton University Press.

Hoad, Neville. 2007. *African Intimacies: Race, Homosexuality and Globalization*. Minneapolis: University of Minnesota Press.
Hodes, Martha. 1997. *White Women, Black Men: Illicit Sex in the 19th-Century South*. New Haven: Yale University Press.
Holland, Sharon Patricia. 2012. *The Erotic Life of Racism*. Durham: Duke University Press.
Holms, Douglas R., and George E. Marcus. 2008. "Cultures of Expertise and the Management of Globalization: Toward the Re-Functioning of Ethnography." In *Global Assemblages*, edited by Ahiwa Ong and Stephen Collier, 235–52. New York: Wiley.
Holsey, Bayo. 2008. *Routes of Remembrance: Refashioning the Slave Trade in Ghana*. Chicago: University of Chicago Press.
Hook, Derek. 2005. "The Racial Stereotype, Colonial Discourse, Fetishism, and Racism." *Psychoanalytic Review* 92 (5): 701–34.
Hudson, Derek. 1972. *Munby: Man of Two Worlds, The Life and Diaries of Arthur J. Munby, 1828–1910*. London: John Murray.
Hunt, Lynn. 1996. *The Invention of Pornography: Obscenity and the Origins of Modernity, 1500–1800*. New York: Zone Books.
Hyam, Ronald. 1990. *Empire and Sexuality: The British Experience*. Manchester: Manchester University Press.
Jean-Baptiste, Rachel. 2014. *Conjugal Rights: Marriage, Sexuality, and Urban Life in Colonial Libreville, Gabon*. Athens: Ohio University Press.
Jones, Hilary. 2013. *The Métis of Senegal: Urban Life and Politics in French West Africa*. Bloomington: Indiana University Press.
Jordan, Mark D. 2015. *Convulsing Bodies: Religion and Resistance in Foucault*. Stanford: Stanford University Press.
Julien, Isaac. 1994. "Confessions of a Snow Queen: Notes on the Making of *The Attendant*." *Critical Quarterly* 36 (1): 120–26.
Katz, Jonathan Ned. 1995. *The Invention of Heterosexuality*. New York: Dutton.
Kaufmann, Jean-Claude. (2010) 2012. *Love Online*. Translated by David Macey. Cambridge: Polity Press.
Kendrick, Walter. 1996. *The Secret Museum: Pornography in Modern Culture*. Berkeley: University of California Press.
Kennedy, Duncan. 1992. "Sexual Abuse, Sexy Dressing and the Eroticization of Domination." *New England Law Review* 26: 1309–93.

Kennedy, Hubert. 1988. *Karl Heinrich Ulrichs, Pioneer of the Modern Gay Movement.* Boston: Alyson.

Kinsey, Alfred C., Wardell B. Pomeroy, and Clyde E. Martin. 1948. *Sexual Behavior in the Human Male.* New York: W.B. Saunders Co.

Köhler, Joachim. 2002. *Zarathustra's Secret.* New Haven: Yale University Press.

Kopytoff, Igor, and Suzanne Miers, eds. 1977. *Slavery in Africa: Historical and Anthropological Perspectives.* Madison: University of Wisconsin Press.

Koven, Seth. 2004. *Slumming: Sexual and Social Politics in Victorian London.* Princeton: Princeton University Press.

Krafft-Ebing, Richard von. (1902, 12th German ed.) 1965. *Psychopathia Sexualis.* Translated by Franklin S. Klaf. New York: Stein and Day.

Krips, Henry. 1999. *Fetish: An Erotics of Culture.* Ithaca: Cornell University Press.

Kulick, Don. 1995. "The Sexual Life of Anthropologists: Erotic Subjectivity and Ethnographic Work." In *Taboo: Sex, Identity and Erotic Subjectivity in Anthropological Fieldwork,* edited by Don Kulick and Margaret Willson, 1–28. London: Routledge.

Kunzel, Regina. 2008. *Criminal Intimacy: Prison and the Uneven History of Modern American Sexuality.* Chicago: University of Chicago Press.

Landes, Ruth. 1940. "A Cult Matriarchate and Male Homosexuality." *Journal of Abnormal and Social Psychology* 35 (3): 386–97.

Latour, Bruno. (1991) 1993. *We Have Never Been Modern.* Translated by Catherine Porter. Cambridge: Harvard University Press.

———. 2005. *Reassembling the Social: An Introduction to Actor-Network-Theory.* Oxford: Oxford University Press.

———. 2010. *On the Modern Cult of the Factish Gods.* Durham: Duke University Press.

Leiris, Michel. (1963) 1992. *Manhood.* Chicago: University of Chicago Press.

Leslie, Charles. 1977. *Wilhelm von Gloeden: Photographer.* New York: Soho Photographic Publishers.

Lim, Eng-Beng. 2014. *Brown Boys and Rice Queens: Spellbinding Performance in the Asias.* New York: New York University Press.

Littlewood, Ian. 2013. *Sultry Climates: Travel and Sex since the Grand Tour.* London: Thistle Publishing.
Lowe, Lisa. 2015. *The Intimacies of Four Continents.* Durham: Duke University Press.
Lyotard, Jean-François. (1979) 1984. *The Postmodern Condition: A Report on Knowledge.* Translated by Geoff Bennington and Brian Massumi. Minneapolis: University of Minnesota Press.
Macey, David. 1993. *The Lives of Michel Foucault: A Biography.* London: Hutchinson.
MacGaffey, Wyatt. 1977. "Fetishism Revisited: Kongo 'Nkisi' in Sociological Perspective." *Africa* 47 (2): 172–84.
———. 1988. "Complexity, Astonishment and Power: The Visual Vocabulary of Kongo Minkisi." *Journal of Southern African Studies* 14 (2): 188–203.
———. 1990. "The Personhood of Ritual Objects: Kongo 'Minkisi.'" *Etnofoor* 3 (1): 45–61.
———. 1993. *Astonishment and Power.* Washington, DC: Smithsonian Institution Press for the National Museum of African Art.
———. 1994. "Notes and Comments: African Objects and the Idea of Fetish." *RES: Anthropology and Aesthetics* 25: 123–31.
MacKinnon, Catharine A. 1989. *Toward a Feminist Theory of the State.* Cambridge: Harvard University Press.
Marcuse, Herbert. (1955) 1966. *Eros and Civilization: A Philosophical Inquiry into Freud.* 2nd ed. Boston: Beacon Press.
Marshall, John. 1981. "Pansies, Perverts and Macho Men: Changing Conceptions of Male Homosexuality." In *The Making of the Modern Homosexual,* edited by Kenneth Plummer, 133–54. London: Hutchinson.
Massad, Joseph. 2002. "Re-Orienting Desire: The Gay International and the Arab World." *Public Culture* 14 (2): 361–85.
Masuzawa, Tomoko. 2000. "Troubles with Materiality: The Ghost of Fetishism in the Nineteenth Century." *Comparative Studies in Society and History* 42 (2): 242–67.
Matory, J. Lorand. 1994. *Sex and the Empire That Is No More: Gender and Politics of Metaphor in Oyo Yoruba Religion.* Minneapolis: University of Minnesota Press.

———. 2003. "Gendered Agendas: The Secrets Scholars Keep About Yoruba-Atlantic Religion." *Gender and History* 15 (3): 409–39.
McClintock, Anne. 1995. *Imperial Leather: Race, Gender and Sexuality in the Colonial Context.* New York: Routledge.
McGlotten, Shaka. 2013. *Virtual Intimacies: Media, Affect, and Queer Sociology.* Albany: SUNY Press.
McIntosh, Mary. 1968. "The Homosexual Role." *Social Problems* 16 (2): 182–92.
Meeker, Martin. 2006. *Contacts Desired: Gay and Lesbian Communications and Community, 1940s–1970s.* Chicago: University of Chicago Press.
Meiu, George Paul. 2008. "Riefenstahl on Safari." *Anthropology Today* 24 (2): 18–22.
———. 2017. *Ethno-erotic Economies: Sexuality, Money, and Belonging in Kenya.* Chicago: University of Chicago Press.
Mercer, Kobena. 1994. *Welcome to the Jungle: New Positions in Black Cultural Studies.* New York: Routledge.
Metz, Christian. 1985. "Photography and Fetish." *October* 34: 81–90.
Meyer, Richard. 2002. *Outlaw Representation: Censorship and Homosexuality in Twentieth-Century American Art.* Boston: Beacon Press.
Miller-Young, Mireille. 2014. *A Taste for Brown Sugar: Black Women in Pornography.* Durham: Duke University Press.
Mitchell, Gregory. 2016. *Tourist Attractions: Performing Race and Masculinity in Brazil's Sexual Economy.* Chicago: University of Chicago Press.
Morris, Rosalind C. 1997. "Thailand, Transnationalism and the Transgression." *Social Text* 15: 53–79.
Morrison, Paul. 1993. "End Pleasure." *GLQ: A Journal of Lesbian and Gay Studies* 1 (1): 53–78.
Morrisroe, Patricia. 1995. *Mapplethorpe: A Biography.* New York: Da Capo Press.
Mullins, Greg. 2002. *Colonial Affairs: Bowles, Burroughs, and Chester Write Tangier.* Madison: University of Wisconsin Press.
Mulvey, Laura. 1975. "Visual Pleasure and Narrative Cinema." *Screen* 16 (3): 6–18.
———. 1993. "Some Thoughts on Theories of Fetishism in the Context of Contemporary Culture." *October* 65: 3–20.

Mumford, Kevin J. 1997. *Interzones: Black/White Sex Districts in Chicago and New York in the Early Twentieth Century*. New York: Columbia University Press.

Murray, Stephen O., and Will Roscoe, eds. 1998. *Boy-Wives and Female Husbands: Studies in African Homosexualities*. New York: Palgrave.

Musser, Amber Jamilla. 2007. "The Literary Symptom: Krafft-Ebing and the Invention of Masochism." In *Mediated Deviance and Social Otherness: Interrogating Influential Representations*, edited by Kylo-Patrick R. Hart, 287–94. Newcastle: Cambridge Scholars Publishing.

———. 2009. "Reading, Writing, and the Whip." *Literature and Medicine* 27 (2): 204–22.

———. 2014. *Sensational Flesh: Race, Power, and Masochism*. New York: New York University Press.

Nagel, Joane. 2003. *Race, Ethnicity, and Sexuality: Intimate Intersections, Forbidden Frontiers*. New York: Oxford University Press.

Najmabadi, Afsaneh. 2005. *Women with Mustaches and Men without Beards: Gender and Sexual Anxieties of Iranian Modernity*. Berkeley: University of California Press.

Nash, Jennifer C. 2014a. "Black Anality." *GLQ: A Journal of Lesbian and Gay Studies* 20 (4): 439–60.

———. 2014b. *The Black Body in Ecstasy: Reading Race, Reading Pornography*. Durham: Duke University Press.

Newell, Stephanie. 2006. *The Forger's Tale: The Search for Odeziaku*. Athens: Ohio University Press.

Newmahr, Staci. 2011. *Playing on the Edge: Sadomasochism, Risk, and Intimacy*. Bloomington: Indiana University Press.

Newton, Esther. 1972. *Mother Camp: Female Impersonators in America*. Chicago: University of Chicago Press.

———. 1993. *Cherry Grove, Fire Island*. Boston: Beacon Press.

———. 1996. "My Best Informant's Dress: The Erotic Equation in Fieldwork." In *Out in the Field: Reflections of Lesbian and Gay Anthropologists*, edited by Ellen Lewin and William L. Leap, 212–35. Urbana: University of Illinois Press.

Nguyen, Vinh-Kim. 2005. "Uses and Pleasures: Sexual Modernity, HIV/AIDS, and Confessional Technologies in a West African Metropolis." In *Sex in Development: Science, Sexuality, and Morality in*

Global Perspective, edited by Vincanne Adams and Stacy Leigh Pigg, 245–68. Durham: Duke University Press.

Nyamnjoh, Francis. 2011. "Cameroonian Bushfalling: Negotiation of Identity and Belonging in Fiction and Ethnography." *American Ethnologist* 38 (4): 701–13.

Nye, Robert A. 1993. "The Medical Origins of Sexual Fetishism." In *Fetishism as Cultural Discourse*, edited by Emily Apter and William Pietz. Ithaca: Cornell University Press.

Nyeck, S. N., and Marc Epprecht. 2013. *Sexual Diversity in Africa: Politics, Theory, Citizenship.* Montreal: McGill-Queen's University Press.

O'Higgins, James, and Michel Foucault. 1983. "Sexual Choice, Sexual Act: An Interview with Michel Foucault." *Salmagundi* 58–59: 10–24.

Oosterhuis, Harry. 1997. "Richard von Krafft-Ebing's 'Step-Children of Nature': Psychiatry and the Making of Homosexual Identity." In *Science and Homosexualities*, edited by Vernon A. Rosario, 67–89. New York: Routledge.

Padilla, Mark B., Jennifer S. Hirsch, Miguel Muñoz-Laboy, Robert E. Sember, and Richard G. Parker, eds. 2007. *Love and Globalization: Transformations of Intimacy in the Contemporary World.* Nashville: Vanderbilt University Press.

Paul, Robert A. n.d. "Stereotypes and Prototypes." Paper presented at the 1995 Meeting of the Society for Psychological Anthropology.

———. 2015. *Mixed Messages: Cultural and Genetic Inheritance in the Constitution of Human Society.* Chicago: University of Chicago Press.

Pettinger, Alasdair. 1993. "Why Fetish?" *New Formations* 19: 83–93.

Pierre, Jemima. 2013. *The Predicament of Blackness: Postcolonial Ghana and the Politics of Race.* Chicago: University of Chicago Press.

Pierre, José, ed. (1990) 1992. *Investigating Sex: Surrealist Discussions.* Translated by Malcolm Imrie. London: Verso.

Pietz, William. 1985. "The Problem of the Fetish, I." *RES: Anthropology and Aesthetics* 9: 5–17.

———. 1987. "The Problem of the Fetish, II: The Origin of the Fetish." *RES: Anthropology and Aesthetics* 13: 23–45.

———. 1988. "The Problem of the Fetish, IIIa: Bosman's Guinea and the Enlightenment Theory of Fetishism." *RES: Anthropology and Aesthetics* 16: 87–124.

———. 1993. "Fetishism and Materialism: The Limits of Theory in Marx." In *Fetishism as Cultural Discourse*, edited by Emily Apter and William Pietz, 119–51. Ithaca: Cornell University Press.

———. 1995a. "The Spirit of Civilization: Blood Sacrifice and Monetary Debt." *RES: Anthropology and Aesthetics* 28: 23–38.

———. 1995b. "Capitalism and Perversion: Reflections on the Fetishism of Excess in the 1980s." *positions* 3 (2): 535–63.

Piot, Charles. 2010. *Nostalgia for the Future: West Africa after the Cold War.* Chicago: University of Chicago Press.

Plummer, Kenneth, ed. 1981. *The Making of the Modern Homosexual.* London: Hutchinson.

Poole, Deborah. 2005. "An Excess of Description: Ethnography, Race, and Visual Technologies." *Annual Review of Anthropology* 34: 159–79.

Povinelli, Elizabeth A. 2006. *The Empire of Love: Toward a Theory of Intimacy, Genealogy, and Carnality.* Durham: Duke University Press.

Povinelli, Elizabeth A., and George Chauncey. 1999. "Thinking Sexuality Transnationally: An Introduction." *GLQ: A Journal of Lesbian and Gay Studies* 5 (4): 439–50.

Pratt, Mary Louise. 2008. *Imperial Eyes: Travel Writing and Transculturation.* 2nd ed. New York: Routledge.

Preston, John. 1983. *Mr. Benson: A Novel.* San Francisco: Cleis Press.

Puar, Jasbir Kaur. 2002. "Circuits of Queer Mobility: Tourism, Travel, and Globalization." *GLQ: A Journal of Lesbian and Gay Studies* 8 (1/2): 101–37.

Ratele, Kopano. 2006. "Kinky Politics." In *Re-Thinking Sexualities in Africa*, edited by Signe Arnfred, 139–54. Uppsala: Nordiska Afrikainstitutet.

Ray, Carina E. 2015. *Crossing the Color Line: Race, Sex, and the Contested Politics of Colonialism in Ghana.* Athens: Ohio University Press.

Reay, Barry. 2002. *Watching Hannah: Sexuality, Horror and Bodily De-formation in Victorian England.* London: Reaktion Books.

———. 2010. *New York Hustlers: Masculinity and Sex in Modern America.* Manchester: Manchester University Press.

Reid-Pharr, Robert F. 2001. *Black Gay Man: Essays.* New York: New York University Press.

Reiss, Albert. 1961. "The Social Integration of Peers and Queers." *Social Problems* 9: 102–20.

Robinson, Paul A. 1969. *The Freudian Left: Wilhelm Reich, Geza Roheim, Herbert Marcuse.* New York: Harper.
———. 1976. *The Modernization of Sex: Havelock Ellis, Alfred Kinsey, William Masters, and Virginia Johnson.* Ithaca: Cornell University Press.
Rocke, Michael. 1996. *Forbidden Friendships: Homosexuality and Male Culture in Renaissance Florence.* New York: Oxford University Press.
Rosario, Vernon A. , ed. 1997. *Science and Homosexualities.* New York: Routledge.
Rubin, Gayle. 2011. *Deviations: A Gayle Rubin Reader.* Durham: Duke University Press.
Rubin, Gayle, with Judith Butler. 1994. "Sex Traffic: Interview." *differences* 6 (2–3): 62–99.
Rush, Dana. 2013. *Vodun in Coastal Bénin: Unfinished, Open-Ended, Global.* Nashville: Vanderbilt University Press.
Sante, Luc. 1995. "The Unexamined Life." *New York Review of Books,* November 16, 42–47.
Schick, Irvin Cemil. 1999. *The Erotic Margin: Sexuality and Spatiality in Alteritist Discourse.* London: Verso.
Schmidt, Heike Ingeborg. 2008. "Colonial Intimacy: The Rechenberg Scandal and Homosexuality in German East Africa." *Journal of the History of Sexuality* 17 (1): 25–59.
Schneider, David. 1980. *American Kinship: A Cultural Account.* 2nd ed. Chicago: University of Chicago Press.
Scott, Darieck. 1994. "Jungle Fever? Black Gay Identity Politics, White Dick, and the Utopian Bedroom." *GLQ: A Journal of Lesbian and Gay Studies* 1: 299–321.
———. 2010. *Extravagant Abjection: Blackness, Power, and Sexuality in the African American Literary Imagination.* New York: New York University Press.
Scott, Joan W. 1991. "The Evidence of Experience." *Critical Inquiry* 17 (4): 773–97.
Sedgwick, Eve Kosofsky. 1985. *Between Men: English Literature and Male Homosocial Desire.* New York: Columbia University Press.
———. 1990. *Epistemology of the Closet.* Berkeley: University of California Press.

Sedgwick, Eve, and Adam Frank. 1995. "Shame in the Cybernetic Fold: Reading Silvan Tomkins." *Critical Inquiry* 21 (2): 496–522.

Shaw, Gwendolyn Dubois. 2004. *Seeing the Unspeakable: The Art of Kara Walker.* Durham: Duke University Press.

Shaw, Rosalind. 2002. *Memories of the Slave Trade: Ritual and the Historical Imagination in Sierra Leone.* Chicago: University of Chicago Press.

Shelton, Anthony. 1995. "The Chameleon Body: Power, Mutilation and Sexuality." In *Fetishism: Visualising Power and Desire,* edited by Anthony Shelton, 11–52. London: South Bank Centre and Brighton: The Royal Pavilion, Art Gallery and Museums.

Simon, William. 1996. *Postmodern Sexualities.* London: Routledge.

Smith, Daniel J. 2007. *A Culture of Corruption: Everyday Deception and Popular Discontent in Nigeria.* Princeton: Princeton University Press.

Smith, James Howard, and Ngeti Mwadime. 2014. *Email from Ngeti: An Ethnography of Sorcery, Redemption, and Friendship in Global Africa.* Berkeley: University of California Press.

Smith, Michael J. 1983. *Black Men White Men: A Gay Anthology.* San Francisco: Gay Sunshine Press.

Spring, Justin. 2010. *Secret Historian: The Life and Times of Samuel Steward, Professor, Tattoo Artist, and Sexual Renegade.* New York: Farrar, Straus and Giroux.

Stanley, Liz, ed. 1984. *The Diaries of Hannah Cullwick: Victorian Maidservant.* New Brunswick, NJ: Rutgers University Press.

Stein, David, with David Schachter. 2009. *Ask the Man Who Owns Him: The Real Lives of Gay Masters and Slaves.* New York: Perfectbound Press.

Stephens, Michelle-Ann. 2014. *Skin Acts: Race, Psychoanalysis, and the Black Male Performer.* Durham: Duke University Press.

Stoler, Ann Laura. 2010. *Carnal Knowledge and Imperial Power: Race and the Intimate in Colonial Rule.* Berkeley: University of California Press.

Stoller, Robert J. 1979. *Sexual Excitement: Dynamics of Erotic Life.* New York: Pantheon.

Stone, Lawrence. 1992. "Libertine Sexuality in Post-Restoration England: Group Sex and Flagellation among the Middling Sort in Norwich in 1706–07." *Journal of the History of Sexuality* 2 (4): 511–26.

Suganuma, Katsuhiko. 2012. *Contact Moments: The Politics of Intercultural Desire in Japanese Male-Queer Cultures.* Hong Kong: Hong Kong University Press.

Sulloway, Frank J. 1992. *Freud, Biologist of the Mind: Beyond the Psychoanalytic Legend.* Cambridge: Harvard University Press.

Tamale, Sylvia. 2011. *African Sexualities: A Reader.* Cape Town: Pambazuka Press.

———. 2013. "Confronting the Politics of Nonconforming Sexualities in Africa." *African Studies Review* 56 (2): 31–45.

Taussig, Michael. 1980. *The Devil and Commodity Fetishism in South America.* Chapel Hill: University of North Carolina Press.

Thompson, Mark. 1991. *Leather Folk: Radical Sex, People, Politics, and Practice.* Boston: Alyson.

Tomkins, Silvan. 1995. *Shame and Its Sisters: A Silvan Tomkins Reader.* Edited by Eve Kosofsky Sedgwick and Adam Frank. Durham: Duke University Press.

Traub, Valerie. 2013. "The New Unhistoricism in Queer Studies." *PMLA* 128 (1): 21–39.

Treat, John. 1999. *Great Mirrors Shattered: Homosexuality, Orientalism, and Japan.* New York: Oxford University Press.

Vance, Carole. 1989. "Social Construction Theory: Problems in the History of Sexuality." In *Homosexuality, Which Homosexuality?*, edited by Dennis Altman, Carole Vance, Martha Vicinus, Jeffrey Weeks, et al., 13–34. London: Gay Men's Press.

Walker, Kara Elizabeth. 1995. *Look Away! Look Away! Look Away!* Exhibition catalogue. Annandale-on-Hudson, NY: Center for Curatorial Studies, Bard College.

Walther, Daniel Joseph. 2008. "Racializing Sex: Same-Sex Relations, German Colonial Authority and *Deutschtum.*" *Journal of the History of Sexuality* 17 (1): 11–24.

Ward, Jane. 2015. *Not Gay: Sex between Straight White Men.* New York: New York University Press.

Waugh, Thomas. 1996. *Hard to Imagine: Gay Male Eroticism in Photography and Film from Their Beginning to Stonewall.* New York: Columbia University Press.

Weeks, Jeffrey. 1977. *Coming Out: Homosexual Politics in Britain, from the Nineteenth Century to the Present.* London: Quartet Books.
———. 1985. *Sexuality and Its Discontents: Meanings, Myths and Modern Sexualities.* London: Routledge and Kegan Paul.
———. 1998. "The 'Homosexual Role' After 30 Years: An Appreciation of the Work of Mary McIntosh." *Sexualities* 1 (2): 131–52.
———. 2005. "Remembering Foucault." *Journal of the History of Sexuality* 14 (1/2): 186–201.
Weinberg, Martin S., ed. 1976. *Sex Research: Studies from the Kinsey Institute.* New York: Oxford University Press.
Weinberg, Martin S., Colin J. Williams, and Charles Moser. 1984. "The Social Constituents of Sadomasochism." *Social Problems* 31 (4): 379–89.
Weinberg, Thomas S. 1987. "Sadomasochism in the United States: A Review of Recent Sociological Literature." *Journal of Sex Research* 23 (l): 50–69.
Weinberg, Thomas, and G.W. Levi Kamel. 1983. *S and M: Studies in Sadomasochism.* New York: Prometheus Books.
Weiss, Margot. 2011. *Techniques of Pleasure: BDSM and the Circuits of Sexuality.* Durham: Duke University Press.
White, Edmund. 1993. *Genet: A Biography.* New York: Alfred A. Knopf.
Wiegman, Robyn. 2015. "Eve's Triangles, or Queer Studies Beside Itself." *differences* 26 (91): 48–73.
Wiegman, Robyn, and Elizabeth A. Wilson. 2015. "Introduction: Anti-Normativity's Queer Conventions." *differences* 26 (l): 1–25.
Williams, Eric. 1944. *Capitalism and Slavery.* Chapel Hill: University of North Carolina Press.
Williams, Erica Lorraine. 2013. *Sex Tourism in Bahia: Ambiguous Entanglements.* Urbana: University of Illinois Press.
Zack, Naomi, ed. 1997. *Race/Sex: Their Sameness, Difference, and Interplay.* New York: Routledge.

INDEX

African and European contact zones, 18–19, 34, 60, 84–85
African and European lovers, 20–23, 44, 52–54, 58, 61–64, 80, 82, 88, 91–93
African origin of fetishes, 12–13, 27, 34–39, 52, 84–85, 95
African slavery: capitalism, 98–99; descent, 69–70; eroticism, 7; extraversion as response, 51–52; golf, 61–62; sadomasochism, 75; slave castles, 23; slave market, 84
antifetish, 40–41
antifetishism, 12

Balibar, Étienne, 101n1
Barthes, Roland, 57-58, 110n4
Bataille, Georges, 50–51, 52, 56
Bayart, Jean-François, 51–52
Bazin, André, 96
Berlant, Lauren, 78
Bersani, Leo, 10, 110n3
Binet, Alfred, 28–29, 31

Blier, Suzanne, 35-36, 52, 101n1
Bloch, Iwan, 1, 109n2
Bowles, Paul and Jane, 4, 90, 93
Burroughs, William, 4
Burton, Sir Richard, 1–2
Byron, Baron George Gordon (Lord Byron), 3–4

Casement, Roger, 60
Chauncey, George, 19, 94, 101n2, 107n7, 108n4
Chester, Alfred, 90
Cole, Jennifer, 81
contact zones: Atlantic African and European, 18–19, 34, 60, 84–85; and cultural boundaries, 91, 109n1; definition, 16; influence of Internet, 90, 95; Japanese and whites, 109n1; love triangles, 93
Cullwick, Hannah, 8, 103n9, 110n2

Davidoff, Lenore, 8
Davidson, Arnold, 32, 47-48, 106n2

desire: Christianity and, 24; contrasted with love, 78; economic bisexuals, 105n5; economics of, 81–82; eroticism, 62–63; fetishes, 15, 30, 105n1, 106n4; long-term relationships, 64; mimetic, 93–94; photographs, 96; prisons, 108n4; racism, 15–16; reproduction, 50; specialization of, 19–20; unexpected, 2; unity, 109n1

Duggan, Lisa, 107n7

Ebron, Paulla, 5
Edelman, Lee, 107n8
Ellis, Havelock, 32
Epprecht, Marc, 102n6
eroticism: African slavery, 7; behavior, 44; capitalism, 8, 97–98; contact zones, 19, 90, 95; definition, 8–11, 13–14, 50–51, 86–87, 89; desires, 62–63; dominance/submission, 69; fetishes, 10, 13–14, 15, 31, 38, 88–89, 97; male-female, 81; money, 97; objectfication, 15; pleasure, 49; politics, 112n3; race, 56, 62–63, 67, 72–73; sexuality, 86–87; social transformations, 47; violence, 110n3
excitement, 8, 41, 65, 69, 85–88, 94, 99
extraversion, 51–52, 53, 59, 70, 91–92

factish, 12, 101n1
Fanon, Frantz, 5, 54, 109n1
fetishes: African origin, 12–13, 27, 34–39, 52, 84–85, 95; body parts, 11, 14, 38-40, 46–47, 79, 88, 107n5, 111n5; capitalism, 8, 29, 97–99; commodities, 21, 29–30, 38, 104n14; definition, 11–12, 28–31, 104n16, 105n1, 109n5; dehumanization, 88–89, 97–98; desire and pleasure, 106n4; eroticism, 10, 13–14, 15, 31, 38, 88–89, 97; feminism, 105n5; and love, 89; military, 40–41; money, 29, 81–82, 97–98; Munby-Cullwick case, 8; pathologies of, 32; photography, 96-97, 110nn2, 4; postcolonial capitalism, 8, 97–98; power, 14–15, 54; racial, 21, 54–59; reaction to, 70–71; social transformations, 20, 39–40, 53, 85. *See also* sadomasochism, sexuality
Fisher, Gary, 112n3
Forster, E.M. (Edward Morgan), 4, 60
Foucault, Michel, 4, 14, 47, 48-49, 94-95, 103n12, 108n3
free and bound, 11–12, 13, 98–99
Freeman, Elizabeth, 84, 112n4
Freud, Sigmund: and Bruno Latour, 104n16; "disavowal" definition, 106n3; feminism, 107n5; modernist fetish definition, 11–12; Oedipal triangle, 93–94; and postmodernist fetish, 106n2; power of fetish, 14–15, 29–30, 85, 88; sadomasochism, 71; *Three Essays on the Theory of Sexuality*, 31–32, 47–48

Gagnon, John, 85, 98
Garber, Marjorie, 94
gay liberation, 10, 42, 108n1
Gebbard, Paul, 71, 111n4
ghetto: African and European lovers, 20–23, 44, 52–54, 58, 61–64, 80, 82, 88, 91–93;

African sexuality, 49;
American, 73; influence of
   Internet, 23–24, 97
Gide, André, 4
Gilman, Sander, 107n5, 109n1
Girard, René, 93–94
Gloeden, Baron Wilhelm von, 2,
   3, 17, 93
golf, 60–62, 63
Graeber, David, 104n14
Guyer, Jane, 33

Halley, Janet, 14, 102n4, 109n5
Halperin, David, 2–3, 83–84, 90, 95
Hart, Keith, 24-25, 106n9
Harvey, David, 19
Hirschfeld, Magnus, 40–41
Hirschman, Albert, 13, 112n1

informal economy, 24-25, 106n9.
   See also unemployment

Julien, Isaac, 7, 84, 112n4

Kinsey, Alfred C., 9-10, 103n12
Kongo *minkisi*, 35–37
Krafft-Ebing, Richard von, 29,
   31-32, 65, 71, 111n4

Lacan, Jacques, 14-15, 106n4
Latour, Bruno, 12, 85, 104n16
Lawrence, T.E. (Thomas Edward),
   4, 60
leather communities, 22, 40-42,
   71-76, 110nn2, 3, 111nn4, 5, 6
love: among prisoners, 49;
   contrasted with desires, 78;
   cultural construction of, 80–81;
   economics of, 104n19; and
   fetishes, 89; influence of Internet,
   19–20; male-male, 1, 4, 5, 92–93;
   Western theory, 15, 104n19

love triangles, 93–94
Lyotard, Jean-François, 30

McClintock, Anne, 8, 103n9
MacGaffey, Wyatt, 35–36
McIntosh, Mary, 43, 108n3
Mapplethorpe, Robert, 57-58, 63,
   110nn2, 3, 111n5
Marx, Karl, 11, 14, 21, 29-31, 85,
   98-99, 101n1
Marxism, 19, 30, 104n16, 108n2
masculinity, 5, 7, 11, 41-42, 55, 72,
   91, 111n3
master-slave erotics, 64, 66-68,
   72-73, 74-77, 111n6, 112n3
Matory, J. Lorand, 92–93
Mediterranean sexual norms, 1-5,
   102n3
Meiu, George Paul, 5
Mercer, Kobena, 57
Metz, Christian, 96–97
Mitchell, Gregory, 97, 104n18
modernist fetishes, 11–12
Munby, Arthur and Hannah
   Cullwick, 8, 103n9, 110n2

nationalism, xv, 96
Newmahr, Staci, 67–70
Newton, Esther, 71, 104n15
Nietzsche, Friedrich, 4
Nyamnjoh, Francis, 52

Orton, Joe, 4

para-ethnography, 59–60, 82
Paul, Robert A., 10, 56, 95-96,
   103n13, 109n1
perversions, 1, 47, 106n2, 107n9
phallus, 29-30, 52, 57-58, 107n5
Pietz, William, 12, 28, 34-36, 38,
   106n1
Piot, Charles, 106n7

postmodernist fetishes, 11-12, 32, 85, 106n2
Povinelli, Elizabeth, 13, 19
Pratt, Mary Louise, 16
Preston, John, 72–73

racism, 15–16, 54–58, 82, 86
Reid-Pharr, Robert, 7
Reiss, Albert, 46
Riefenstahl, Leni, 6, 110
Rubin, Gayle, 70, 97, 103n11, 110n2, 111n4

Sacher-Masoch, Leopold von, 71
Sade, Marquis de, 13–14, 71
sadomasochism: African, 66–67, 69–71; African Internet education, 22; definition, 67–69; leather communities, 22, 40-42, 71-76, 110nn2, 3, 111nn4, 5, 6; masculinity, 7; master-slave erotics, 64, 66-68, 72-73, 74-77, 111n6, 112n3; opposition to reproduction, 47; play scene, 65–66; Sigmund Freud, 71; social transformations, 32
scams, 6–7, 20, 22–23, 52, 63, 66, 76–77, 80
scandal, 1, 101n2
Scott, Darieck, 7
Scott, Joan, 46
Sedgwick, Eve, 90, 94, 102n5, 112n3
sexuality: African, 43–45; behaviors, 103n12; definition, 8-10, 27, 47-49, 83–84, 108n5; eroticism, 86–87; and feminism, 108n2; freedom, 46–47; gender roles, 103n10; media, 95–97; normative, 106n2; power, 62; prisons, 108n4; restriction, 104n18; social transformations, 94–95; spatial boundaries, 90
shame, 5, 70, 87, 97, 98-99, 112n3
Simon, William, 85–87, 96, 98
slavery, 13, 65, 69-70, 74. *See also* African slavery; master/slave erotics
sodomy, 3, 18–19, 75
Steward, Samuel, 32, 41, 73-74, 110n3
Stoller, Robert, 86–89, 98
Stone, Lawrence, 56
Stuart-Young, John, 21, 105n3

teleology and human reproduction, 9-11, 29, 32, 47, 50–51, 104n13, 106n2, 107n8
Tomkins, Silvan, 46-47, 69, 79, 99, 102n5
transgressions, 13, 23, 51, 56

Ulrichs, Karl Heinrich, 4, 102n4, 107n7
unemployment, 22, 24

Walker, Kara E., 7, 99–100
Warhol, Andy, 30
Weeks, Jeffrey, 10, 108n3
Wilde, Oscar, 4
Williams, Eric, 98

www.ingramcontent.com/pod-product-compliance
Ingram Content Group UK Ltd.
Pitfield, Milton Keynes, MK11 3LW, UK
UKHW021811310326
469532UK00005B/173